The Power of Ashtanga Yoga

The Power of
ASHTANGA YOGA

Developing a Practice
That Will Bring You Strength,
Flexibility, and Inner Peace

Kino MacGregor

SHAMBHALA
Boulder · 2013

Shambhala Publications, Inc.
4720 Walnut Street
Boulder, Colorado 80301
www.shambhala.com

14 13 12 11 10 9 8 7 6

Printed in the United States of America

♾ This edition is printed on acid-free paper that meets the
American National Standards Institute z39.48 Standard.
♻ Shambhala Publications makes every effort to print on recycled paper.
For more information please visit www.shambhala.com.

Distributed in the United States by Penguin Random House LLC
and in Canada by Random House of Canada Ltd

Designed by Steve Dyer

Library of Congress Cataloging-in-Publication Data

MacGregor, Kino
The power of ashtanga yoga: developing a practice that will bring
you strength, flexibility, and inner peace/Kino MacGregor
Pages   cm
ISBN 978-1-61180-005-0 (pbk.: alk. paper)
1. Ashtanga yoga. I. Title.
RA781.68.M32 2013
613.7'046—dc23
2012038267

This book is an offering to every sincere student of yoga.
I dedicate this book to my teachers Sri K. Pattabhi Jois
and R. Sharath Jois, to my parents for their constant
support, and to my husband who will always be my hero.
Special thanks to John Miller for awesome photos,
Jack Forem and Greg Nardi for editing, and my agent
Bob Silverstein—without your hard work and faith in me
this book would not exist.

CONTENTS

Acknowledgments   ix

Introduction: How to Use This Book   xi

PART ONE: THEORY

1. Getting Started with Ashtanga Yoga History
   and Tradition   3
2. Heart of the Method: Breath, Pose, and Gaze   19
3. The Ashtanga Yoga Diet   35
4. The Spiritual Journey of Asana: Yoga beyond
   Bending   45

PART TWO: PRACTICE

5. Sun Salutation: Where It All Begins   57
6. Standing Poses: Build Your Foundation   67
7. Seated Poses: Grow Your Lotus   95
8. Backbends: Open Your Heart   137
9. Finishing Poses: Entering the Inner Space   147
10. Strength: The Yoga of True Power   171

Appendix A: Mantras   185
Appendix B: Sanskrit Vinyasa Count   187
Appendix C: The Complete Ashtanga Yoga Primary Series   201
Glossary   211
Resources   217

ACKNOWLEDGMENTS

I CONSIDER IT TRUE GRACE AND GOOD FORTUNE THAT I met Sri K. Pattabhi Jois and his grandson R. Sharath Jois when I had been practicing Ashtanga Yoga for less than a year. Always joyful to see a new student, Jois beamed with the true joy of a man who has touched the heart of yoga. It was his contagious laugh, forgiving grace, unparalleled urgency, and depth of wisdom that gave me faith to practice Ashtanga Yoga six days a week over the last twelve years through pain and injury and into healing. Whenever I studied with Jois as he traveled and taught Ashtanga Yoga around the world, I felt the unique blend of peaceful happiness emanating from his heart. Over the ten years I spent training with him, I always saw him full of energy, love, and enthusiasm for his students. There will never be another teacher or person exactly like him, and we should not seek to replace him. Instead, I hope only to continue practicing and teaching the tradition of yoga that I was lucky enough to receive from him.

I thank my first Ashtanga Yoga teachers, Ryan Spielman and Govinda Kai. I also had the support of my mom and dad, who recognized the healing power of yoga in my life and believed in my dream of sharing yoga with the world. My husband has been a constant source of teaching, evolution, and love. Throughout my journey into Ashtanga Yoga, I have had many angels who guided my way, and I bear a torch of gratitude to everyone who has been a teacher to me. I would not have the legacy of Ashtanga Yoga to share with you if it were not for the generation of Ashtanga Yoga teachers who first traveled to Mysore in the 1970s when I was just a baby. It is because people like Tim Miller, Nancy Gilgoff, and David Swenson dedicated their lives to Ashtanga Yoga that I was able to find it as early as I did.

The journey of a spiritual seeker never ends, and the best teachers always have the open minds of new students. But no matter how much support and help you have, the spiritual journey is a lonely quest that must be walked alone; you are directly accountable for each step you take in any direction. It is your own strength that you discover along the way, and no one but you can truly find that.

IF, INSTEAD OF READING THIS PAGE, YOU WERE SITTING with me in a practice room at my South Beach, Florida, wellness center, the first thing I'd say would probably be, "Welcome! Thanks for coming today." Because I'd be happy to see you and because yoga is my life and my passion, I'm always grateful for the chance to share it.

I'd also probably say, "Congratulations for doing this," whether it's your first step into the world of yoga or the next step to deepening and enriching your ongoing practice. I know from my own experience and that of my students that regular, daily practice leads to real and lasting peace. It is a path lit by the torch of your own consciousness, guarded by a lineage of teachers that starts with the sages of India's historic past and culminates in the millions of people who practice yoga today. When your body, mind, and soul come to rest in the sacred movements of yoga, you join an international community dedicated to living life fully at peace. The real magic of yoga lies not in any specific movements but in its universal ability to transform the lives of its practitioners — including you. So I welcome you today and congratulate you for your good fortune (or perhaps, good karma) in discovering and embracing this transformative knowledge.

MY YOGA JOURNEY

Like many Americans, I was introduced to yoga at a gym. When I was nineteen and more interested in fitness than spirituality, I noticed that some of my fellow aerobicizers attended the gym's yoga class; they had more defined arm muscles and were able to do headstands. This piqued my curiosity. Observing the class, I couldn't make much sense of the stretching, breathing, and bending. Yet something within me was drawn to these somehow-familiar movements. So I decided to try.

Back then, I had no idea that there were different types of yoga, but I know now that the first class I took was from the Sivananda tradition. Focusing on gentle stretches, relaxation, and deep breathing, this class was calm, peaceful, and (to my young and restless mind) totally boring. So boring, in fact, that I never went back. But something about it had resonated with me, because when I injured both of my Achilles tendons about a month later, I turned to yoga to help me heal. I had no clue that I was about to reconnect with my inner self and begin a lifelong journey.

My injury was so debilitating that I had a hard time walking without the support of air casts. The sports medicine doctors I consulted recommended surgery. Instead I bought books on yoga from the Sivananda tradition and other Hatha Yoga schools, canceled my gym membership, and began the slow road to recovery that has taken more than a decade. This road became a pathway of discovery that involved far more than just physical health. The practice of yoga provided me with such profound emotional and spiritual healing that I have devoted my life to sharing this remarkable, transformative tradition.

The series of poses in this book are an accessible introduction to the lineage of Ashtanga Yoga that I learned directly from my teachers, Sri K. Pattabhi Jois and R. Sharath Jois. I hope you are inspired to begin your own yoga practice at home and then continue under the guidance of a qualified teacher. I am honored to be your guide for this initiation to the yoga that has changed my life so completely, and I hope you will join me on the yoga journey, which is ultimately the journey to yourself.

With the wisdom gained through true self-awareness, you will come to know yourself deeply, directly, and powerfully. With regular daily practice, you will see your body transform, feel more energetic, and actually be happier and more compassionate.

No matter how often you practice these movements, you will never get to the end of your yoga journey. If you have looked ahead at some of the pictures or had a chance to watch any of the DVDs in which I demonstrate the various levels of Ashtanga Yoga, you may feel there is no way you will ever be able to accomplish these poses. I could easily have said that when I first started. But I hope you will be inspired to give it your best shot, remembering that all yoga teachers and advanced practitioners were once beginners. We all had our doubts, our moments of wanting to quit, our pain and fatigue. But we kept going, and that is the great lesson and the great achievement. The eternal wisdom of yoga places emphasis not on perfection of the asanas for their own sake, but on the state of equanimity achieved after many years of devoted practice. Achieving that inner calm and balance is fueled by your inspiration, dedication, heart, and soul.

THE HEART OF ASHTANGA

It wasn't just the life-changing injury that propelled me to look more deeply at yoga. I wanted a way out of the pain and suffering of my past. I felt lost and alone in the world and did not know anyone or anything that helped me find a direction for my life. My body cried out for health and healing, my heart yearned for a more peaceful life, and the only thing I felt I could turn to was yoga.

Joining a class at a yoga center seemed to carry a whole new depth of commitment, much more than a yoga class at a gym or following pose sequences out of a book at home. As I walked through the courtyard that led to the Miami Beach center where I took my first Ashtanga Yoga class, I was transported into an alternate reality. A small fountain bubbled gently, and incense wafted through the open doors. I bought a drop-in class for fifteen dollars, rented a yoga mat for a dollar, and took my postgym competitiveness into the practice room for a proper schooling.

The friendly people at the front desk directed me through the doors to the yoga room. Exotic, unfamiliar statues and flowers in a vase on an altar that held photos of Indian men had me wondering what on earth I was getting myself into. I was in totally new territory, unsure of myself and excited at the same time. Then the instructor arrived, and his dark curls and soft-spoken manner disarmed me as he asked if I had ever tried Ashtanga Yoga before. When I said that I hadn't, his response of "Well, do what you can" and a slightly sardonic smile made me doubt that I had indeed made the right decision in joining this class.

Just as the inner cynic inside me was about to win the debate, roll up the rental yoga mat, and go home, the teacher began the class by intoning, "OM." We hopped on the Ashtanga Yoga train, and it didn't stop for nearly two hours. Thinking myself relatively fit despite my injured ankles, I thought I would be fine. Little did I know how weak, stiff, and uncoordinated I was until I tried getting through that class! From the start, when I attempted my first Sun Salutation, I bellyflopped my way through the push-up poses and floundered around like a fish out of water. I couldn't lift my body weight off the ground, steady my mind, breathe freely, touch my toes from standing, or accomplish any of the other movements the teacher made seem so effortless. Halfway through the class, I saw another student hoist his hips off the ground from a seated position and enter a half-handstand. I felt like I was watching the circus. When I tried it, I felt like my body was permanently glued to the ground. I couldn't even catch an inch of air.

By the time we got to the headstand, I was desperate; my arms were shaking, and I didn't have an ounce of strength left. The teacher came and gave me a pass, instructing me to rest. I was never so thankful to anyone!

When we were finally finished, I was lying in a pool of my own sweat. Yet I remember feeling truly happy and free for the first time in my life. My mind cleared, my breathing deepened, a soft smile crossed my lips, and a pulsing sensation arose in the base of my spine and traveled all the way to the top of my head. My soul seemed to have an answer to questions it had been asking for years. My heart felt at home in my own skin. I walked out and purchased my first yoga mat and a class card good for ten yoga sessions. I practiced every Tuesday and Thursday until I moved to New York City to complete my graduate studies at New York University.

After my move, I joined a traditional Mysore-style Ashtanga Yoga practice group. The first week that I practiced six out of seven days, as the tradition recommends, I was so sore that I couldn't lift a glass of water without my arms shaking. I had to rest my elbow on the edge of the sink to put on my mascara. But it was wonderful, because I was really feeling my body's innate potential for the first time. It was like graduating to a new level of yoga, and I loved every moment of it.

In New York, I learned that this tradition of yoga was taught by the then-living master Sri K. Pattabhi Jois, who lived in a small city in South India called Mysore (Karnataka). I read his book, *Yoga Mala,* every night before bed. I wanted to let his wisdom and knowledge sink deeply into my psyche, so I took my time, reading and digesting each word. The night I finished reading the book, I dreamed of Jois although I hadn't yet met him. I woke up with the words "I have to go to India" on my lips. I bought my ticket two weeks later. Instead of completing the New York internship I had planned for the two-month summer break, I found myself on the first of many trips to India.

When I arrived in Mysore, far from my own culture, I had no idea what to expect. A student of 2001 academe, I was skeptical of the idea of a guru. The nearly thirty-hour journey took me across two continents, through three airports, and down old dirt roads where cows wandered freely. A taxi finally dropped me off at the Ashtanga Yoga Nilayam in the old neighborhood of Lakshmipuram. I walked up the steps to the back-alley entrance and found Sri K. Pattabhi Jois teaching a group of twelve sweaty yogis; many more were waiting their turn. He turned, looked me in the eyes, and asked if I was there to practice. Before doubt surfaced, my heart opened. I fell to my knees, saying, "Yes, I'm here to practice. Thank you, Guruji." I knew I had met my teacher—not only because I had seen him in a dream but because his very presence opened my heart, eased my pain, and brought me peace. From that day forward, I called him Guruji, an honorific title that students use to indicate acceptance of their teacher as their spiritual guru. For the remainder of this book, I will refer to him as Jois for the sake of clarity, but in my heart, he will always be Guruji.

Jois's teaching—that each student must work the sometimes arduous path of Ashtanga Yoga to find lasting peace — resonated with me. He never promised to be a magical healer. Instead, he always said that he was just a simple man teaching the yoga that his teacher, Sri T. Krishnamacharya, had taught him and always stressing that yoga is for everyone.

It never occurred to me that I would be a yoga teacher. When I was a little girl, I dreamed of being a Supreme Court justice, a politician, or some force for social change in the world. Much to my surprise, after my first trip to India, people started asking me to teach. Though I felt unworthy and tried to direct these inquiries toward instructors I believed were more qualified, people persisted in asking me, so I began to teach. During my second trip to India in 2002, a fellow practitioner with a yoga center in Ireland invited me to lead a workshop. I was both honored and shocked, and I humbly accepted. Today, my husband and I own a yoga center in South Beach, and I travel the world sharing the tradition of yoga that has changed my life. Every day when I walk into the center we have built, I smell the fragrance of nag champa incense and feel the welcoming atmosphere created by hundreds of students who practice there every week.

I have been teaching Ashtanga Yoga for about twelve years. My annual teaching schedule takes me to about thirty-five cities in twenty countries, in addition to my regular classes in Florida. So it is no exaggeration to say that I have worked with thousands of students of all ages and at all stages of practice — from absolute beginners to advanced practitioners — throughout North and South America, Asia, and Europe. I have also, of course, put in many thousands of hours of personal practice, advancing slowly but surely from that first eye-opening class to ever-higher levels of proficiency. From my own and my students' experience, I am well aware of the difficulties, doubts, and frustrations that you may sometimes encounter as you begin your journey, but I'm also aware of the ever-greater mental clarity, emotional balance, energy, and happiness that you will feel as you continue.

The practice of yoga is a decision to believe in yourself against all odds. It is a choice you make to walk down a self-empowering path toward your own liberation from suffering. As you train your mind to remain steadfast, you unravel cycles of misery and follow a path that leads toward true freedom. My childhood dream to leave the world a more peaceful place comes true every time I share Ashtanga Yoga with sincere students. I hope that you will take the gift of practice and allow it to transform your life too.

PRACTICAL GUIDELINES FOR YOGA PRACTICE

Ashtanga is a vigorous, sweat-producing style of yoga that purifies your body from the inside out. Three points of attention create the foundation for the practice: yoga poses (asanas), yogic breathing techniques, and a

Getting Started in Your Practice

- It is ideal to practice yoga first thing in the morning on an empty stomach. If you need to practice later in the day, try not to eat for at least two hours beforehand.
- Wear clothes that you can sweat in, and practice on a flat, even surface.
- Use a yoga mat that feels right for you. It is important that you buy a personal yoga mat. Using your own mat is more sanitary than renting one at a yoga center, and it will accumulate your spiritual energy. Choose a mat that is manufactured from ecologically sustainable materials that will not break down too quickly.
- You will probably need at least a small hand towel while you practice to wipe the perspiration off your face. If you sweat profusely, you will need a larger towel to place over your yoga mat.
- Wear comfortable clothes that are appropriate for exercise—nothing

specific gazing point for each movement. The poses are arranged sequentially so that each pose builds on the previous one in ever-increasing levels of difficulty. Ideally, you should learn one pose at a time directly from a teacher. If you are practicing on your own, it is important that you give yourself time to learn the full sequence slowly rather than jumping ahead to poses that look like fun or trying to do all of the poses at once. You will have the best results if you build your healing practice from the beginning to the end and allow yourself to become acclimated to each new movement and place careful emphasis on breathing deeply rather than on the perfection of physical form. If you can't resist the temptation to skip ahead to poses that are beyond your present level of experience, I strongly advise you not to just look at the pictures and try the movements; rather, it would be best if you read all of Part One before proceeding to the chapters on practice. Regardless of whether you attempt only the Sun Salutation or try the full practice, you will generate the detoxifying sweat that this method is known for.

Ashtanga Yoga is more than just an exercise routine; it is a body awareness technique that helps you experience deeper levels of peace, increased energy, better health, and greater happiness. At all stages of your yoga journey, remember to listen to your body and respect your limitations whether they are physical, mental, or emotional. The inner journey cannot be rushed, and one of yoga's greatest lessons is that of patience and acceptance. If you are in extreme discomfort at any time, relax and back off a little, knowing that you have eternity to learn exactly what you need to learn. You should never experience pain in your joints when you practice yoga. At the same time, you want to challenge yourself just enough to expand your consciousness and transform your body. If you are a total beginner, you can expect to experience a little muscle soreness after trying these poses for the first time; that's normal, so allow yourself to enjoy the feeling of working your body in a safe, tested, and proven way.

OVERVIEW OF THE BOOK

This book is divided into two sections: theory and practice. The four chapters on theory provide the historical and philosophical foundation for Ashtanga Yoga.

Chapter 1 is an account of the method's history and tradition, including the story of my teacher, Sri K. Pattabhi Jois. I also share a bit of my own story and personal discovery of Ashtanga Yoga.

Chapter 2 goes into greater detail about the three fundamental points of the method — breath, pose, and gaze. My teacher often said that Ashtanga Yoga is meant to teach students how to breathe and that the rest is really just bending. Without the breath, he said, there is no yoga. The central gazing point, called *drishti* in Sanskrit, is meant to train the mind to remain centered on a single point of attention. The three-pronged approach of Ashtanga Yoga, called the Tristana method, guides your daily discipline.

Chapter 3 outlines the benefits of a yogic diet for the health of both the individual practitioner and the planet as a whole. Built on the principle of nonviolence, yoga philosophy recommends that devoted students model their eating habits on peaceful principles and asks that they consider a vegetarian diet. Taking responsibility for all the products you consume, including food, is part of a lifestyle commitment to inner and outer peace.

Chapter 4 sets the foundation for what I consider my most important message: yoga is a spiritual path leading toward enlightenment, or true and lasting inner peace.

Section Two addresses the physical practice of Ashtanga Yoga. It breaks down the complex method pose by pose in an accessible, user-friendly format that includes illustrations and instructions on how to perform the asanas at home. A chapter is devoted to each of the five groups of poses in the Ashtanga Yoga Primary Series: the Sun Salutation, standing poses, seated poses, backbends, and finishing poses.

If you are new to yoga, attempt only one chapter at a time and follow the beginner's guidelines. Once you become proficient at the asanas in one chapter, you may safely proceed to the next, until you can do the entire sequence together. Try starting with about twenty minutes of practice each day and build up as you add more poses; it may take you several years to be able to complete a full hour-and-a-half practice. If you are already familiar with the Ashtanga Yoga Primary Series, the chapters will give you a detailed guide to alignment, technique, and the history of the poses.

Throughout this book, I will show you how Ashtanga Yoga practice connects the physical with the spiritual in a way that leads to lasting transformation. When you unroll your yoga mat and commit to the total journey of yoga, you unlock the mind's power to transform physical substance with the power of spirit.

There is no sense of entitlement on the path. To maintain both belief and effort over a sustained period of time, you will need to tap into a place inside yourself that is beyond the physical. Grace in yoga is earned through devoting yourself to achieving higher consciousness and ultimately becoming a force of healing in the world. Proficiency on the journey of yoga takes time and dedication. It is not a quick fix, but all the benefits that you experience will be lasting and true.

too loose or too tight. Choose clothes that provide a good level of support yet are easy to move in, such as a cotton/lycra blend.

- You will get the best results if you treat this practice like a daily healing ritual. If possible, dedicate a space in your home entirely to your yoga practice.

- You may find that lighting a small candle and a stick of incense helps create a sense of sacred space, which all yoga practice really deserves.

- Start each practice session by consciously dedicating yourself to yoga and your inner journey.

- After practicing these asanas at home for a while, you will find it beneficial to seek the guidance of a teacher who can tailor your practice to your unique abilities and needs. When looking for a teacher, consult published lists of qualified instructors, research the local centers where you wish take classes, and ask other students for recommendations.

PART ONE

Theory

1

Getting Started with Ashtanga Yoga History and Tradition

If we practice the science of yoga, which is useful to the entire human community and which yields happiness both here and hereafter — if we practice it without fail, we will then attain physical, mental, and spiritual happiness, and our minds will flood toward the Self.

— *SRI K. PATTABHI JOIS*

WHILE THE SPIRITUAL BENEFITS OF YOGA ARE CENTRAL to this ancient path, the physical aspect is what draws most students. It is certainly true practicing yoga leads to better health, less stress, and a happier, more peaceful mind. But while it may be tempting to think of yoga as merely another exercise routine, its real healing benefits come from its integrated approach to working with the body and mind.

Modern research has discovered what the yoga tradition of India has known and relied on for thousands of years: the mind and body are intimately connected. In fact, they are one continuum. The body may be viewed as the physical expression of the mind and spirit. Thus, when you think and act in a habitual way, thought patterns take root in the mind and translate into physical conditions in the body. Chronic stress, unhealthy eating patterns, low cardiovascular function, low immune function, prolonged feelings of anxiety, and many other conditions associated with our modern lifestyle can be treated and healed with regular yoga practice. Yoga poses work to literally change the mind's established patterns, replacing negative networks and pathways in the brain with healthy, happy patterns. Bending and moving the body in new ways encourage the mind to operate in a manner that is more conducive to long-term well-being.

"Over seventy-five scientific trials have been published on yoga in major medical journals. These studies have shown that yoga is a safe and effective way to increase physical activity that also has important psychological benefits due to its meditative nature."

—*Steffany Haaz, MFA, RYT*[1]

Here are some of the scientifically proven benefits of yoga:

- Increases flexibility and agility
- Promotes better balance
- Increases feelings of well-being and improves body image
- Regulates high blood pressure (hypertension)

---

1. Steffany Haaz, "Yoga for People with Arthritis," The Johns Hopkins Arthritis Center, last updated June 23, 2009, www.hopkinsarthritis.org/patient-corner/disease-management/yoga-for-arthritis.

The mere practice of the asanas has a healing effect. Forward bends purify the midsection of the body of any excess fatty tissue and help to optimize digestive function. Twisting the torso wrings out the body like a towel from the inside, encouraging the digestive system to work more efficiently and facilitating the removal of stored weight. The gentle pressing of the organs helps any accumulated toxins find their way out of the body. The combination of cleansing poses and deep breathing increases the body's capacity to renew itself. The breath acts as another mechanism for the removal of old toxins and waste materials while calming and clarifying the mind.

Deep breathing has a direct effect on the nervous system. Part of the magic of yoga practice stems from its reliance on the power of breath regulation. While performing the asanas, you are mindful of your breath and regulate it carefully using specific techniques that lengthen and deepen your breathing. A long, slow, steady breath is associated with the relaxation response, a mind-body state associated with health and healing. (We will discuss this in detail in Chapter 2.)

Listening to the Wisdom of Your Body

Yoga poses give you a chance to access the spiritual through the physical. This process of internal awakening makes it possible for dedicated practitioners to excavate layers of themselves. Each physical pose presents an opportunity to heal the body and train the mind; through practice, yogis develop a more deeply attuned way of living, being, and acting.

Yoga is a sanctuary where you learn to listen to your body. Like a holiday from the limiting and often negative thoughts that run on autopilot at the back of your mind, the focused stillness of yoga opens a space for you to appreciate the true nature of your mind. When your capacity to listen is at its greatest and most refined, you can listen directly to your soul and seek its constant guidance.

Paying careful attention to and sensing the inner body allows yoga practitioners a daily opportunity for reflection. By regularly tuning in to this internal level, yogis become increasingly aware of the alignment or misalignment of their actions in daily life. The body's wisdom lies in its pervasive truthfulness, and the yogi's wisdom lies in the willingness to listen to the body's sometimes superior sense of itself. It clearly reveals its physical and spiritual story. Through years of dedicated practice, students of yoga learn to distinguish true inner messages from fanciful whims and desires. They learn to walk a delicate tightrope between healthy guidance and destructive old habits that are hard to change.

The Ancient Origins of Yoga Poses

To understand how the asanas are part of a true spiritual tradition rather than merely a fitness routine, you will need at least some knowledge of the historic tradition of asana as a spiritual practice in India. The earliest known reference to yoga is found in the Pashupati seals, which were used by the Indus Valley civilization more than three thousand years ago. These seals depict human forms in yogalike poses similar to Baddha Konasana from the Ashtanga Yoga Primary Series and Mulabhandasana, or Root Lock Posture, from the Ashtanga Yoga Fourth Series.

The Vedas are India's oldest spiritual texts, dating from 3000 to 1200 B.C.E., and they contain practical guidelines for attaining metaphysical experiences. The term *asana* appears in a yogic context in the Atharva Veda Samhita (1500 B.C.E.) and in cosmogonic myths that describe ascetics with folded legs and soles turned upward as in Padmasana; it is a reference to divinity entering the body. The Vedas were a layered and textured way of performing rituals to maintain consonance between the individual, society, and the cosmos. The Atharva Veda is magical in nature, whereas the Rig, Sama, and Yajur Vedas are more about the rituals and poetry that seek to codify the ecstatic experience.

The next period of Indian philosophical thought, dating from 900 to 500 B.C.E., is detailed in the Upanishads (which literally means "to sit near," referring to the need to learn at the feet of a true teacher). These texts focus on discovering the truth behind reality and attaining liberation from suffering. The Upanishads represent an evolution from the Vedic culture, and although the earlier texts don't mention yoga, they describe protoyogic thought and technique. The *Katha Upanishad* is the first to use the word *yoga* specifically in reference to the careful training of the mind and body to be absolutely one-pointed and still inside. It states, "This they consider to be Yoga: the steady holding (*dharana*) of the senses. Then one becomes attentive (*apramatta*); for Yoga can be acquired and lost" (*Katha Upanishad* 2.3.11, translation by Georg Feuerstein).

It may be helpful to make a distinction between the evolution of yoga theory and that of yoga asana. Asana is not fully representative of yoga as a whole, and there is more evidence regarding yoga's development than there is of the development of asana. While asana developed within the context of the larger philosophy and theory of yoga, it would be incorrect to say that they are the same. Asana is a subset of yoga and one — perhaps foundational — step in the full eight-limbed path of Ashtanga Yoga.

Yoga poses as a practice appear in the epic period of Indic thought as evidenced in the Mahabharata, which mentions two asanas — Mandukasana (Frog Pose) and Virasana (Hero Pose). The Mahabharata details an epic

- Reduces pain, including that caused by chronic back problems, arthritis, carpal tunnel syndrome, and osteoporosis
- Helps relieve depression
- Reduces stress
- Reduces tension, anxiety, and worry
- Helps relieve premenstrual and menopausal symptoms
- Benefits the heart and increases cardiovascular function
- Increases immunological and digestive function
- Elicits the relaxation response

Yoga practice has many other advantages that have not yet been systematically studied. These include weight loss, help with eating disorders, better sleep, more energy, heightened awareness, increased capacity for empathy, and regulation of brain waves.

battle between good and evil, written in the format of a dialogue between King Dhritarashtra and Sanjaya. The section known as the Bhagavad Gita is a dialogue between Krishna and Arjuna that precedes an eighteen-day battle on the field of Kurukshetra. In the Bhagavad Gita, authored by Vyasa, Krishna as the avatar of the god Vishnu teaches the warrior prince Arjuna the yoga of perfect actions, the yoga of perfect devotion, and the yoga of perfect knowledge. The *Yoga Yajnavalkya* (200 B.C.) describes Padmasana (Full Lotus Pose), Simhasana (Lion Pose), and Mayurasana (Peacock Pose) and distinguishes between physical poses for purification and meditative poses for spiritual realization.

Around the second century B.C.E., during India's Mauryan empire, Patanjali compiled the four books of the Yoga Sutras, which are dedicated to the practice of yoga. Patanjali defines yoga as the concentration of the mind on a single point of attention, clearly outlines the full eight-limbed path of Ashtanga Yoga, and identifies the practice of asana as the third limb of this path. This yoga philosophy integrates previous notions of sacrifice (*yajna*) with personal practice in the concept of *tapas,* the acceptance of pain that leads to purification. Tapas, translated literally as "heat," was a precursor to physical yoga practice. Severe austerities were the means of purification, leading to the awakening of internal fire into which sacrifices are made. The original vedic ritual was the *homa* or fire sacrifice. Agni is a deity seen as a messenger of the gods; through Agni, offerings into the fire would be delivered to the realms of the gods. In Patanjali's system, *asana* means a meditation seat of which only a few practitioners are considered worthy. In the *Yoga Bhasya* (the first commentary on the Yoga Sutras), Vyasa lists thirteen asanas, all of which are meditative sitting poses. Patanjali says that asana should be steady and comfortable and that a practitioner should relax his or her effort while focusing on the infinite. However, out of his 196 aphorisms on yoga only a few relate directly to asana practice. Most of Patanjali's text outlines the philosophical tenets of spiritual practice. There is speculation that asana was passed on from teacher/guru to student so that specific instructions on pose were only given directly by the teacher, but this cannot be verified. Another theory is that the lack of attention to asana in the text indicates either the inferior position that asana plays in the yogic journey or its preparatory nature for the spiritual journey. The eight-limbed path outlined in Patanjali's Yoga Sutras describes the ultimate goal of yoga as final liberation through the steady cultivation of practice and nonattachment, and asana plays a vital role. Some scholars suggest that the first book of the Yoga Sutras (*Samadhi Pada*) lists the means of practice and nonattachment for advanced practitioners who have already controlled their senses and established a *sattvic,* or peaceful, mind. According to them, the second book (*Sadhana Pada*) lists the eight limbs of Ashtanga Yoga for those who are still working to establish the foundations of deeper practice.

The last millennium produced multiple treatises on asana as a physical practice. Perhaps the most influential is the *Hatha Yoga Pradipika* (1400 C.E.), which outlines numerous yoga asanas with detailed descriptions of the technique and the spiritual benefits. Its author, Swami Swatmarama, firmly claims that the practice of yoga poses in combination with breathing practice and concentration on a single point of attention leads to final liberation from the cycle of suffering. All physical yoga practice of the current era can be said to fall under the banner of Hatha Yoga. The *Yoga Upanishads* (1500 C.E.), the *Shiva Samhita* (1700 C.E.), and the *Gheranda Samhita* (1800 C.E.) detail even more yoga poses and continue Patanjali's principles.

There is nothing to say that Hatha Yoga is not an expansion of Patanjali's system, but there are definitely significant differences. While the *Hatha Yoga Pradipika* states that Hatha Yoga is a ladder for reaching Raja Yoga, the Yoga Sutras do not identify Patanjali's system as Raja Yoga. Neither Hatha Yoga nor Raja Yoga is specifically mentioned in the Yoga Sutras, but the foundational elements of both can be found in Patanjali's text. It is commonly assumed either that they are synonymous or that Raja Yoga comprises the last three "inner limbs" of Ashtanga Yoga. Either way, they are related but distinct paths. My teacher often said that the last three limbs of the Ashtanga Yoga system are internal. While this might seem confusing, Jois's system seems to be a hybrid of the Ashtanga Yoga of Patanjali and Hatha Yoga.

Today's multifaceted yoga continues the constant evolution and dialogue of yoga as a science of spiritual realization grounded in the continuity of daily practice. The Ashtanga Yoga method comes from this ancient spiritual lineage through the expert hands of Sri T. Krishnamacharya and his main students. The next section details the specific history of this method. The spiritual heart of asana practice is the key to the Tristana method of Ashtanga and is discussed in Chapter 2. Without the awareness that all poses have the final liberation of the soul as their intention, the movements are just physical. The poses derive their healing benefits from their ability to access the deepest level of human consciousness.

THE ORIGINS OF ASHTANGA YOGA

The historical origins of Ashtanga Yoga are as much legend as fact. The tradition traces back to an ancient sage named Vamana Rishi. We do not know much about him other than that he is the purported author of the *Yoga Korunta*. Even this legendary text is not available for study, because all of it was destroyed by time and eaten by ants.

The next person in the lineage was Rama Mohan Brahmachari, who lived in a cave on Mount Kailash (in the Himalayas) with his wife and three children. No one knows what happened to his children — where they went or if they became yoga teachers. Rama Mohan Brahmachari taught his student, Sri T. Krishnamacharya, from a copy of the *Yoga Korunta*. Part of the legend is that when it was time for Krishnamacharya to leave his teacher, Rama Mohan Brahmachari instructed him to go out and teach yoga to the world but to tell no one where they could find him.

Krishnamacharya is known as the source of most of the yoga that is now popularly taught in the West. His students included the great teachers B. K. S. Iyengar (who established Iyengar Yoga), Sri K. Pattabhi Jois (Ashtanga Yoga), A. G. Mohan (Svastha Yoga), T. K. V. Desikachar (Viniyoga), Indra Devi, and countless others. Following lineage in yoga is much like tracing a family tree. You learn from a teacher who is a student of a master. That master was once a student of another master. The origins of yoga follow an unbroken line from teacher to student through a nearly five-thousand-year journey in Indian history. Although recent scholarship has questioned the truth of an unbroken lineage of asana practice, the spiritual heart of yoga as the search for inner peace is as old and eternal as the human spirit itself. Preserved without the use of computers, printers, and external hard drives, most yoga knowledge is acquired and passed on through memorization.

Ashtanga Yoga in the tradition of Sri K. Pattabhi Jois is a dynamic form of Hatha Yoga that asks you to unroll your mat a staggering six days a week. It is sometimes so demanding as to be intimidating. When I started practicing Ashtanga Yoga, I was just like you. When I finished each practice, I was sore all over and not particularly good at it. I also did not have the seemingly superhuman strength or the Gumbi-like flexibility that the poses require. But I learned both through years of sincere practice. Many people assume that because they cannot easily bend their bodies into the pretzel-like positions of the Ashtanga Yoga Primary Series that this method is not for them. The sole qualification for the practice of Ashtanga Yoga is to love your practice and to "show up" on your mat as much as possible. It does not matter what level of asana you perform, because the inner work of yoga is fueled by the authentic search for inner peace. If I did it, so can you.

The method I teach in this book comes from the lifework of my teacher who taught for more than seventy years before his death on May 18, 2009. The miracle of Jois's life and legacy far exceeds his physical presence and is perhaps the very definition of the word *guru*. He was born in July 1915 in a small village called Kowshika (South India) on Guru Purnima day, which is designated as an Indian national holiday to honor all gurus. His life embodied the tradition of the sacred teacher-student relationship. Jois discovered yoga at age twelve and was a devoted student when he first saw Sri T. Krishnamacharya, the man who would become his teacher. He continued his education in yoga and Sanskrit studies at the Mysore

University until, after thirty-seven years of professorship, he earned the title of Vidwan (professor emeritus of Sanskrit studies). Jois died when he was ninety-three after dedicating his life to teaching Ashtanga Yoga, which he had introduced to the West. With years of experience teaching in the small South Indian city of Mysore, Jois's unwavering diligence in maintaining the Ashtanga Yoga method as he had learned it from Krishnamacharya allowed thousands — if not millions — of people to benefit from regular practice. Without his steady perseverance, yoga as we know it today simply would not be.

ASHTANGA SPIRITUAL PRACTICE

Ashtanga literally means "eight limbs," which are defined by Patanjali's Yoga Sutras as *yama* (moral codes), *niyama* (self-purification and study), *asana* (pose), *pranayama* (breath control), *pratyahara* (sense control), *dharana* (concentration), *dhyana* (meditation), and *samadhi* (total peace). Ideally, teachers are well versed in their knowledge of all eight limbs before they begin teaching so they may truly guide their students through the entire journey of yoga. Yet the different levels of samadhi are not readily attainable to everyone in a short period of practice — perhaps not even in one lifetime; the method described by Patanjali was reserved for only the highest guru. Some teachers suggest that all physical yoga is merely a preparation for deeper yogic states that can only be experienced in the presence of a fully enlightened master.

Jois taught that regular physical practice cleanses the area around the spiritual heart and removes the six poisons of *kama* (desire), *krodha* (anger), *moha* (delusion), *lobha* (greed), *matsarya* (envy), and *mada* (sloth). These six poisons are called the *arishadvarga,* a term found in the third chapter of the Mahabharata, one of the epics of ancient India, from which Adi Shankaracharya taught. Adi Shankaracharya was the main Indian teacher of nondualism and Advaita Vedanta philosophy, and his work greatly influenced Jois's philosophy on life, spirituality, and the divine. My teacher was a firm believer in daily practice as the main method for practitioners to experience the benefits of yoga. To remove the six poisons, you have to practice with strong determination and change layers of deeply rooted, negative behavioral patterns (*samskaras*) that can only be eradicated through yogic purification. Daily practice of all eight limbs of the Ashtanga Yoga path slowly transforms your mind into a peaceful place.

The yamas are moral codes that tell us how to engage with the world ethically. They include *ahimsa* (nonviolence), *satya* (truthfulness), *asteya* (nonstealing), *brahmacharya* (sexual responsibility), and *aparigraha* (nonattachment). The niyamas are ethical guidelines that define how we should relate with ourselves. They include *sauca* (cleanliness), *santosha* (contentment), *tapas* (heat and purification), *svadhyaya* (spiritual self-inquiry), and *ishvara pranidhana* (devotion to the divine).

When this integrated approach to spiritual development is in place, the inner fire of purification (*agni*) is ignited and literally burns through unhealthy habits, physical toxins, and emotional hang-ups. The agni is said to coincide with the awakening of spiritual energy within the body and is accompanied by tremendous inner heat. It is also associated with the digestive fire. Simply studying and memorizing the Yoga Sutras, Sanskrit terms, or contemporary philosophy will not give you peace. Information alone is not knowledge. Jois always emphasized the necessity of experiencing the true effects of a daily practice within your own body and life. Only in this way can you integrate the wisdom of the sacred, eternal teachings of yoga into your everyday life and know firsthand the empowering self-knowledge that is the essence of yoga. Yoga transforms people not by demanding change but by inspiring it from within, and daily practice provides the foundation for this transformation.

ASHTANGA PHYSICAL PRACTICE

Ashtanga Yoga asks you to work on the spiritual through the physical. You begin by sweating your way through some yoga poses while concentrating your mind on your body, breath, and gaze. The theory that I share with you in this book is largely my own constantly evolving experience rather than an official statement of the Ashtanga Yoga method for all time. It is a mirror that I hope you will use to look deeply within yourself and discover the logic and magic of the method.

Ashtanga Yoga practice is broken up into six groups of poses. The first group, called the Primary Series, is a pretty strenuous routine. Most people will spend their entire lives working on elements of this set of seventy-two poses. Known in Sanskrit as *yoga chikitsa*, this practice cleanses your organs, tissues, and glands of toxins, fat, and other harmful substances. The Primary Series contains all the necessary elements for establishing health and purifying your body, including Surya Namaskara (Sun Salutation), forward bends, twists, backbends, powerful lifting, headstands, and many other movements that stoke the inner fire. The specific nature of Ashtanga Yoga is that you repeat the poses in the same order until you have mastered them. You do not move on until you have made some sort of progress where you are. When you repeat a series of poses over and over, you move away from an intellectual understanding of them to a kinesthetic intelligence that connects movement to a place deep within.

The Ashtanga Yoga Primary Series builds sequentially in terms of flexibility and strength to prepare you for some of the gateway poses in the practice. Gateway poses test a student's understanding of technique and asana. These postures are the most challenging in the set of related poses. Starting with Surya Namaskara, which is aimed at both steadying the mind and warming up the inner fire, the practice lengthens the hamstrings, stretches and strengthens the back, increases core development, and purifies the entire body. Surya Namaskara is where the student of yoga begins to develop devotion (*bhavana*). The gateway posture of the standing poses lies in Utthita Hasta Padangusthasana (Extended Hand-to-Big-Toe Pose) in which you must balance on one leg, lift your other leg, bend forward, suck in your lower belly, and externally rotate your hip joint all in one pose.

Once you can perform this pose easily, it is safe to move on to the next series of poses, which includes the four versions of Marichasana (Pose Dedicated to Sage Marichi). These poses require a series of binds where you clasp your hand either behind your back or around your leg in a twisted pose and maintain either a half-lotus or a very strong extended leg. The careful placement of every asana that precedes this section of the practice is aimed at developing the internal strength and flexibility needed to perform these four poses easily. Marichasana D is the pinnacle of this portion of the series, being the most difficult twist and half-lotus combination.

The grand crescendo of the Primary Series is Supta Kurmasana (Sleeping Tortoise Pose), in which internal strength, external rotation, and forward bending are strongly challenged as you try to get both legs behind your head. After this point, the poses help transition from flexing to extending the spine so you can perform Urdhva Danurasana (Lifted Bow Pose) or other backbends with ease. Backbending is itself a gateway posture that challenges the strength and flexibility of the spine. The logic of the Primary Series builds up to certain poses that test alignment, inner strength, and flexibility to make sure your asana practice is solid and stable before you move on.

The Second, or Intermediate, Series of Ashtanga Yoga is called nerve cleansing (*nadi shodhana*). In this set of even deeper backbends, hip openers, and strength poses, practitioners work on cleaning the nervous system. The Advanced Practice is a balance of strength and grace and is divided into Advanced A/Third Series, Advanced B/Fourth Series, Advanced C/Fifth Series, and Advanced D/Sixth Series. I currently practice Advanced A and B or Third and Fourth Series. Jois used to say that yoga is 99 percent practice and 1 percent theory. The highest form of knowledge for the yoga practitioner is that which has been experienced directly and is therefore rooted in direct faith. The forum for this direct experience is a physical practice of asanas that induce a powerful, cleansing sweat when done regularly. To realize the benefits of yoga, you must practice as much as possible. It is not something that can be explained in philosophy; it is something that must be directly experienced within. With the careful coordination of pose, breath, and concentration, the internal fire of purification ignites and the journey of transformation begins. If you try Ashtanga Yoga, you will soon experience the deluge of sweat and the heat of purification.

The Ashtanga Yoga method recommends that you practice six days a week. Traditionally, this practice was meant to be done in the "Mysore style," in which you follow your own breath and movement rather than the guidance of a teacher leading a class through the same movements. Named after the city in South India where Jois lived and taught, this is the safest and best way to practice. Memorizing the poses allows you to focus internally, which is the real goal of yoga. When you do not know what you will be doing next, your attention will always be on your teacher rather than within yourself. Once you memorize the sequence of poses that your teacher determines is right for you, the entire practice moves to a deeper, subconscious level. Practicing in the Mysore style allows you to go deeply into your practice some days and take it more gently other days, always performing the same poses. This natural variation prevents injury, trains you to listen to your body, and increases internal body awareness. Additionally, Mysore style is the only way to learn the most advanced poses of the six series of Ashtanga Yoga, since few individuals can perform and teach these highly challenging poses.

Taking on a six-day-a-week practice is often hard for new students, so I usually recommend that they begin with three days. Once they establish that level of regularity, they can add one day every six months until they reach the full six days a week. To make the transition from a fitness-oriented approach to yoga to a devotional one, you need to practice consistently and regularly. A daily spiritual ritual in which you take time to connect internally to a deep sense of yourself requires dedication. The six-day requirement is meant to develop the kind of mental, spiritual, and devotional determination needed to progress along the internal path of yoga. If you accept yoga as a lifelong commitment to inner peace, it behooves you to practice as often as you can. If you only practice when it's convenient or when you feel good, then yoga is more of a hobby that you take up and put down at will. But sincere spiritual practice can never be just a leisurely activity if it is to result in awakening. True spiritual practice is an unbroken commitment to do everything it takes to see the deepest truth there is. It is not something you can choose to look at on Monday and Wednesday and pretend it does not exist for the rest of the week.

On a purely physical level, a six-day-a-week practice is both advantageous and challenging. By performing the poses more often, you will see results faster, building strength, stamina, and flexibility at a faster pace than if you were to practice only once or twice a week. In fact, those individuals who choose to attend yoga class once a week are actually setting themselves up for a weekly struggle in which they must always face the same weaknesses and other issues; they have no chance of realizing improvement through sustained practice.

It is no secret that if you do practice six days a week, you will be physically sore. This very soreness is tied to the notion that the acceptance of some pain is good along the path toward purification—the concept of tapas described earlier in this chapter. The idea is that certain pains, such as the pain of releasing an old habit, of cleansing the body, or of letting go of attachments, must be accepted along the road to purification. Tapas can also mean controlling the senses, food, and the body, which ultimately leads to the rise of a sattvic mind. Practicing six days a week accelerates the rate at which you experience the pains that purify weakness and stiffness, as well as the rate at which you experience the purified result of more strength and flexibility in the body and mind.

On many of my trips to Mysore, students would share their elaborate stories of muscular discomfort with Jois, and most of the time he would say, "Pain good." The only way that the inner fire of purification can work is if you learn to stay with it, see it clearly, and not run away. The natural human response to pain is fear, avoidance, and denial, yet yoga uses pain as a method of awakening. Muscular pain in yoga is often felt as burning or shaking and can be accepted, but joint pain is a different teacher, and when it is experienced you should back off. By learning to accept certain pains within the safe space provided by yoga, you learn to create a pause between the pain stimulus and the response in your body and mind that wants to run away. In that powerful pause, you are able to choose your course of action instead of being driven by reactionary patterns from the past. Past experiences leave marks deep within the mind called samskaras. These impressions color future experiences and accumulate to form deep habit patterns in the mind. Once the samskaras aggregate into larger patterns of attraction or aversion, they are known as *vasanas*. Samskaras and vasanas draw us into repetitive loops wherein we repeat past actions, patterns, and events over and over. To a large degree, our samskaras and vasanas determine the course of our future actions and our karma. One form of yoga is actually called Karma Yoga and is the act of being mindful of thoughts and actions in an effort to release samskaras. Samskaras and vasanas can be burned away through yogic meditation techniques. If you truly want to use your yoga practice to whittle away at your sleeping store of negative karma and behavioral patterns, then you must practice as often as possible.

It is important to define practice at this point. To burn through samskaras, the mental practice that accompanies asanas is paramount. *Practice* is defined by Patanjali's Yoga Sutras as the cultivation of a state of samadhi or peace along with the mental state of nonattachment. Asana is presented as one of the ways to actively practice these more esoteric states of being. The result of asana practice is defined in Yoga Sutra 2.48 as freedom from dualities such as pleasure and pain, attachment and aversion. Two of the obstacles to the spiritual path are attachment and aversion that result from the experience of pleasure and pain. The untrained human mind runs toward pleasure and away from pain, and this constant effort fuels the cycle of suffering. Regular asana practice teaches yoga practitioners how to maintain a balanced state of mind and ultimately break free from this addictive pattern.

This promise of inner peace does not come cheap. You cannot beg, borrow, or cheat your way along the inner journey. Creating a new way of being is not simply a matter of flipping a switch. Instead, you stand at the foot of the mountain of new desire and look ahead to a long and sometimes rigorous road to the top. With years of work, patience, and diligence, anything is possible. Yet when faced with such adversity, most people quit or take the easy, known route to average results. While there is nothing wrong with this philosophy, there is a much more powerful way to live your life to its maximum potential. Yoga leads the way through disbelief into an accomplished life.

Within the boundaries of a sticky mat, yoga practitioners repeatedly perform challenging movements while uniting their breath, pose, and gaze. Krishnamacharya described yoga as the process by which the impossible becomes possible and the possible over a long period of time becomes easy. The place where many practitioners fall off the path is when they try to go straight from impossible to easy. If you experience a movement as impossible and want it to be easy immediately, you will certainly fail, because change does not happen quickly. Instead, you need to start with the impossible and allow its difficulty to teach you. Stay in those ugly places where learning happens, and soon the impossible starts to show you how it may one day be possible. Almost no one gets it right on the first try. Held within the outward form of every light, free, and easy pose are years of difficulty, failure, and even pain. When you embark on the inner quest of yoga, it is the very process of starting at the bottom of a seemingly unscalable mountain and climbing it with slow, steady perseverance against insurmountable odds that holds the power of transformation. By conquering the unconquerable and confronting the terrifying places within, you necessarily gain access to an experience of yourself that is beyond the struggle, the experience of a place within yourself that is eternally peaceful, powerful, and loving. That is what yoga is all about. The light, free, and easy asana is just a matter of seduction. Yoga teaches that only by transcending the illusory world of limitations can you actually move past these false boundaries in your practice and in your life. Every pose, every movement, and every breath along the way redefines the very essence of your being.

In a sense, yoga is the most basic path of self-empowerment. The tricky part of the path is that the self that is being empowered is not the ego of

Western psychology. It is the highest Self within, the soul whose direct experience leads to self-transcendence and a death of the small ego. Some people interpret yoga as a practice meant to strengthen the ego, but it is actually meant to burn away the small ego and release the resplendent inner light within.

FINDING YOUR TEACHER

While the tradition of yoga is intimately bound up in the sanctity of the teacher-student relationship, the words and guidance of even the greatest teachers are only meant to be signposts that lead students to the discovery of their own true voice within. Years under a teacher's heartfelt guidance can give you the gift of finding your highest teacher within. No genuine teacher wants students to do what he or she says just because he or she said it or because it is written in some ancient scripture.

When you begin your search for a yoga teacher, look for one whose training comes from a verifiable lineage. Most official schools of yoga, like Ashtanga Yoga, list their teachers online so you can check the listings to find a school close to where you live. Remember that being a good teacher is more than just having a piece of paper that logs in a certain amount of hours. You have to trust your teacher instinctively and be drawn to his or her presence. The best yoga teachers will be able to give you good anatomical and technical direction. Teachers in the Ashtanga Yoga tradition should ideally know the basics of the philosophical tenets of the traditional practice. Yoga schools that pay homage to the sacred tradition usually put their teachers through additional training before allowing them to take students. For example, at my yoga center in Miami, we train all our teachers directly even if they have gone through a training program somewhere else.

Choosing a teacher and a school is not as casual as shopping for the perfect pair of shoes. It is a complex process that ideally employs your body, mind, and spirit. Most important, the teacher must be someone you can trust and believe in to be your guide. Verify his or her qualifications by speaking with older students who have been practicing more than ten years with one teacher to get a feel for how the practice works over a long period of time.

At its best, yoga is a nondogmatic, nonreligious path toward self-realization. All yoga is experiential by definition, because no one can do your daily practice or live your awakening for you. No matter how many times you read about it or hear it from your teacher, nothing on the path is real for you until you actually feel it in your own body, mind, and soul. Teachers and tradition illuminate the path for you, but you have to take each step with your own two feet.

The role of the teacher is traditionally considered an absolute necessity along the spiritual journey; however, many contemporary yoga teachers promote the idea of being self-taught and downplay tradition. The concept of a guru is even harder for many Western yoga students, who are raised in a culture of independence, to understand. Yet in the Indian tradition, the teacher-student relationship is a sacrosanct part of the journey into the inner world.

Ashtanga Yoga is now taught by legions of certified and authorized teachers in more than thirty countries. These teachers include Jois's son, Manju Pattabhi Jois, in California; his daughter, Saraswathi Rangaswamy, in Mysore; and his grandson, R. Sharath Jois, also in Mysore, who is now the head of the lineage. When researching yoga teachers, check to be sure that they have spent sufficient time studying the method either directly in India at the K. Pattabhi Jois Ashtanga Yoga Institute or with other senior Ashtanga Yoga teachers. It would be ideal to make the journey to India yourself or to choose a teacher who is certified or authorized by Sri K. Pattabhi Jois or R. Sharath Jois. If you do not have immediate access to a qualified teacher for daily classes, you can begin your practice at home with the guidance of books such as this one, DVDs produced by qualified instructors, and the wealth of information available online such as www.kpjayi .org and www.ashtanga.com. Then you can augment your home practice by traveling to take a workshop or immersion course and learn the method more completely.

Once your practice of Ashtanga Yoga has sincerely begun, you will need to choose a teacher who will be your main guide in the method. I still remember the magic of my first meeting with Jois in Mysore. It changed my life forever, and it inspires every day that I practice. This is an experience that only your heart can lead you toward, because the inner journey is a sacred space that can only be shared with someone whom you trust and love.

THE HEROIC HEALING JOURNEY OF YOGA

The quiet world of our inner being can sometimes get drowned out by the loud stresses of daily life. Yet when you begin a yoga practice, you open a door to a tranquil space of listening. It is here, in the inner world, where healing takes place. At its most basic level, yoga seeks to reunite you with your deepest understanding of body, mind, and soul. This singular state of consciousness helps you regain the lost world of yourself as you really are: peaceful, free, and beautiful.

Everyone wants to be happy. No matter how different people may seem, everyone wants to know real peace and lasting freedom. By engaging with the enjoyable yet challenging yoga poses, you learn how to conquer obstacles and attain freedom. This may well be the greatest gift that yoga offers its practitioners.

On the inward journey of yoga, every dedicated practitioner encounters beautiful epiphany moments that lead to awakening and transcendental experiences of healing. But every dedicated practitioner also encounters obstacles: laziness, fear, lack of confidence, low self-esteem, the anger born of frustration over poses that seem insurmountably difficult. These obstacles — most, if not all, of them related to deep-rooted patterns — are as formidable and challenging as the demons, tricksters, and tempters of the mythological hero's journey. In the sacred stories of heroic battles, the tests and trials are really opportunities to face the deepest secrets of the self and return free from fear. The obstacles faced by every hero reflect the inner journey. The inward journey of yoga makes every practitioner play the lead role in their own epic saga. When you practice, you have a chance to go on your own quest and become Odysseus in *The Odyssey* or Arjuna in the Bhagavad Gita. From the Buddha to Luke Skywalker in *Star Wars,* one factor that unites every mythological hero's journey is that transformation contains the seeds of a dramatic spiritual awakening. And just as the heroes of the great myths ultimately faced their challenges alone, each student of yoga is ultimately responsible for winning his or her own freedom.

Each of my eleven trips to India was a chapter in my inner adventure, in which I observed ever more deeply the true nature of spiritual strength. On my first trip, I was humbled to see how far I had to go to realize both the physical strength and the steadiness of mind that the spiritual path demands. Under the careful guidance of my teacher, I was able, after years of dedicated practice, to tap into an eternal place within from which all strength flows. Since I was not naturally strong or able to perform the more challenging poses of Ashtanga Yoga, I had to unearth a sleeping strength far beyond anything I ever imagined possible. Every challenging arm balance, handstand, and backbend was a microcosm for the transformation of my soul. The Ashtanga Yoga method is deceptively simple. You may read about the principles and think you understand them, but only after many years of practice have I begun to realize just how powerful the practice really is.

2

Heart of the Method:
Breath, Pose, and Gaze

WHEN I FIRST TRAVELED TO MYSORE, JOIS TOLD ME to focus on three simple things: breath, pose, and gaze. Called the Tristana method, these three points form the basis of Ashtanga Yoga. While it is crucial to follow the entire eight-limbed spiritual path of Ashtanga Yoga outlined in Chapter 1, to realize a full physical and spiritual transformation and to attain inner peace, the Tristana method gives practical guidelines for safely performing the asanas.

The most prevalent aspect of today's yoga tradition is the practice of poses, which have a deeply healing effect. Each pose is discussed in great detail in Part Two of this book. Forward bends encourage practitioners to bend and release inside the pelvis, thereby purifying the torso of any excess fatty tissue and optimizing digestive function. Twisting poses wring out the body like a towel from the inside, encouraging the digestive system to work more efficiently and gently pressing the internal organs to help move any accumulated toxins out of the body. However, no pose alone has a healing effect. Practicing the asanas while breathing deeply increases the body's capacity to renew itself. Holding your mind steadily on a single point of attention first trains the mind to be one-pointed and then leads to a steady focus on the inner body. Only with all three components of the Tristana method will you experience the transformative power of Ashtanga Yoga.

HOW THE YOGA POSES REALLY WORK

The healing benefit of the physical practice of yoga is as easy to understand as the benefit of brushing your teeth every day. When you use your body on a daily basis, sediment accumulates along the interior spaces. If you never clean out this store of toxins and impurities, the body will begin to decay. Yoga poses cleanse the body from within by going into the darkest corners with twists, bends, folds, and breath to literally burn through stuck material. Without the constant cleansing of asanas, the internal workings of the body's organs and neuromuscular systems grow sluggish. But with a regular yoga practice, the body is able to maintain a healthy level of pliability throughout life. The Ashtanga Yoga method in particular leaves no cell untouched and systematically brings strength and flexibility to the entire body.

On an emotional and psychological level, the yoga poses increase conscious awareness of every part of the body. Along with the pure physical benefit associated with this heightened awareness, numerous mental and emotional benefits accrue as well. Just like plaque accumulates on the teeth and inside the arteries, old emotions remain stored within the subtle body. The physical body is closely related to the subconscious mind. When you delve deeply into sleeping areas of the body, you discover that the body itself is a reservoir of old memories, emotions, and habits. The samskaras, or negative habit patterns of the body and mind, take root in the body and manifest in postural patterns such as tightness, stiffness, and pain. When yoga poses force you to go directly into the source of the old habit pattern and face the fear, sadness, anger, or other traumatic emotions, they are providing the deepest therapy possible. With yoga practice, you can release and cleanse old mental and psychological blockages that have taken root deep within your subtle body. Without ever needing to know why these emotional patterns are there or where they came from, yoga frees you from the past and opens your mind to a lighter, brighter future.

The asanas work first on a practice level to burn through the toxins in the physical, emotional, and energetic bodies. The poses also work to change the basic hardwiring of the mind. Normally, when we confront difficult situations, we want to run away. If we encounter a scary memory, we often want to bury it. This pattern, while totally natural, is not effective at creating a truly happy, healthy life. Yoga trains the mind to stay in places of difficulty instead of running away and developing protective measures. In yoga, there is no room for defense mechanisms. In fact, the yoga poses are designed to strip away every protective layer you may have developed to reveal the inner purity at the heart of your being. When a particularly deep samskara is triggered during your practice, you may find yourself in the midst of a deep emotional release. Without warning, you may suddenly feel vulnerable, start crying, shake with fear, tremble with anger, or experience many other intense emotions. The main difference between yoga and psychotherapy is that you never need to ask or know why something is happening. All you have to do is experience it directly and fully. While you will certainly cleanse your consciousness of the scars and wounds of the past, the best gift yoga gives you is the retraining of the mind's habit patterns to help you face difficulty directly with a brave heart.

DRISHTI: SINGLE-POINTED GAZE

When I first started practicing, I failed to fully grasp the importance of *drishti,* or a single gazing point. I felt that if I was able to maintain a pose, that was enough. I remember being in the yoga shala in Mysore and allowing my mind to wander so I could see what was going on around me. I was interested in what my teacher was doing with other students, what poses other students were doing at different levels of proficiency, what kind of clothes people were wearing, what type of yoga mats were most popular, and who was waiting in line to practice next. I focused least on the inner body. It was the epitome of an untrained mind. Each time I returned to Mysore, my teacher would strongly remind me of the importance of drishti by reiterating that it is key to the mind training of yoga. In his broken English, Jois would teach more through presence than verbose explanations. It took me at least four trips to India before I really understood that no drishti means a weak mind, and a weak mind means no yoga is happening. I did not have a naturally strong mind, but the diligent practice of drishti helped me connect with a one-pointedness of perception that exceeds anything I thought I could accomplish.

In Ashtanga Yoga, each pose has a specific gazing point; the place where you are directed to focus your eyes plays an important role in the spiritual development of your practice. *Drishti* literally means "vision" or "insight," and its purpose is to direct the gaze to a focal point of attention and influence both what you see and your way of seeing. The mind is reflected in the gaze, so the point where your mind rests during yoga practice will determine the ultimate success of your effort along the path. In essence, drishti practice endeavors not just to bring your eyes to a random point but also to train your mind to be centered within a spiritual paradigm. Directing the mind to a single point of attention prevents your thoughts from wavering and focusing on the external; it simultaneously helps you practice the strength and steadiness of mind to remain one-pointed, which is an important goal of all yoga practice.

Practically speaking, drishti is an essential tool for finding balance while physically moving. Balance is a state of mind that is expressed through physicality. You cannot find physical balance while your eyes are darting around the room. Yoga generally assumes that the practitioner's state of mind is reflected in his or her physical practice. The mind directs the body; it also directs the eyes to gaze toward the points of most salient interest. The gaze then directs the energy or intention of the practitioner. A gaze directed at one of the drishtis instills a deep inner practice, whereas a gaze directed at many fluctuating external points fosters an unsteady, unfocused mind. In essence, if the student's eyes are wandering, then so is the mind. If the student's eyes are focused on a single object, then the mind too remains calm and attentive. Only a calm, clear mind can strip away the layers of ego, old habit patterns, pain, and ignorance to reveal the brilliant light of consciousness.

There are nine drishtis in Ashtanga Yoga, and each presents an opportunity for a different inner realization:

- Gazing between the eyebrows (*broomadhya drishti*) opens the third eye (*ajna*) chakra and encourages energy to rise up the spine through the central column of the body, toward the center of the head where the seat of spiritual knowingness resides.
- Gazing upward (*urdhva* or *antara drishti*) helps continue the careful movement of energy up the spine so that the life force can rise and awaken spiritual centers within the brain.
- Nose gazing (*nasagrai drishti*) closes the eyes slightly, thereby limiting the amount of optical stimulation received from the external environment and encouraging the power of sight to be directed inward. Gazing at the tip of the nose also slightly crosses the optic nerve, which — when done successfully — opens the central channel of the brain (the corpus callosum) and harmonizes deep brain activity along both hemispheres.
- Navel gazing (*nabi chakra drishti*) stimulates the solar plexus (the *manipura* chakra), helps direct the mind toward the inner body, and encourages a subtle flexing of the spine.
- Gazing toward the fingers or toes (*hastagrai drishti* or *padhayoragrai drishti*) directs your energy through space, giving the physical body a sense of boundlessness. These two drishtis also play an important role in maintaining a sense of balance while performing the physical asanas.
- Gazing toward the thumb (*angustha ma dyai drishti*) helps students find balance by bringing their attention to the end point of certain poses. It extends the energy of the pose outward from the center and stimulates the meridian points in the thumb, which are traditionally thought to be symbolic of fire, similar to that of purification that all Ashtanga Yoga seeks to kindle. The thumb is also a symbol of the cosmic divine, and the connection of the thumb and index finger in certain poses is said to symbolize the individual consciousness uniting with the divine.
- Gazing to the left or right (*parsva drishti*) concentrates the mind on the more subtle flow of energy in the body and helps perfect the physical pose. When a student is able to maintain the drishti in a relaxed, open, and free manner during the practice of physical asana, it is generally an indication of integration and mastery of that particular pose.

Only during final relaxation, called Sukhasana (Easy Pose), do the eyes remain closed. Jois would often joke that if you close your eyes during asana practice, sleep would come soon. Without the specific points of attention, asana practice would lose some of its intensity and not be as successful at effecting the kind of spiritual and psychological transformation that is its ultimate goal.

Gazing with the Lamp of Knowledge

The etymological roots of the word *drishti* can be traced back to the Sanskrit *drs,* which literally means "to see," as in the power of conscious sight. More than mere casual sight, this root word implies that the act of seeing includes the light of spiritual understanding. Another common derivation of *drs* is *drsya,* or the light in which all objects present themselves to the higher intelligence of each individual being. Similarly, the root *drs* yields *drastr* (the seer), known as the *purusha,* or individual soul within every sentient being. Historically, the drishti plays an important part in the conscious redirection of the mind toward spiritual understanding. The word *dhrik-sthiti* is found in the *Tejo Bindu Upanishad* (1.29) as one of the practices of the fifteen-fold path. It is defined as that wise vision that sees the world as the Absolute and must not be confused with mere gazing at the tip of the nose. The *Mandala Brahmana Upanishad* (2.26) identifies three types of drishti during meditation: eyes open, eyes half-open, and eyes closed. The definition of *dhrik-sthiti* is reminiscent of my teacher's definition of *pratyahara* — wherever you look, you see God. When the light of inner understanding is directed toward specific points of attention within the body during yoga practice, students directly experience their true nature within.

By directing the power of sight to the inner body, asana practice opens a door to the experience of one of the more subtle limbs of the Ashtanga Yoga path. When the powers of the sense organs are directed away from the external world and toward the inner body, you experience sense withdrawal. Defined in Sanskrit as *pratyahara,* it is also the fifth limb of the Ashtanga Yoga method. Without the ability to redirect your attention away from the seductive external world, the mind will always be called out of spiritual realization into sensory experiences. The purpose of yoga is to prepare the mind and soul for ultimate freedom from the seemingly endless cycle of experiences. Only when the mind can actually stay focused on one point of attention for a sustained period is it possible for it to perceive deeper levels of reality. Drishti is one practice that trains the mind to be both singular and subtle in its point of attention.

Yoga practice is the methodical retraining of the mind to be focused on spiritual realization. First students learn to maintain one-pointed gaze and then later develop single-pointed attention. This single-pointed attention (*ekagrata*) demands that the practitioner have a strong, steady mind. The Mahabharata states that "the singleness of the senses is the highest form of tapas" (12.242.4). The practice of ekagrata prevents the mind from attaching itself to one object, one person, or one thought by staying intently focused on the divine. While performing physical asanas, the calm, clear mind takes precedence over any fantastic feat of pose. One way to ensure that your priority is spiritual development is to place careful emphasis on the drishti in every pose. A common definition of yoga is the ability to maintain a singular point of attention. The object of attention is chosen at will, and the evidence of a trained mind is the sustained concentration on a certain point with unwavering focus. Drishti is a tool that every yoga practitioner can easily use to train the mind to remain steady and strong, thereby increasing peaceful, calm feelings.

The ultimate goal of all yoga practice is the single-pointed revelation of the divine soul within. The practice of drishti allows students to develop the spiritual paradigm that leads to wisdom, often defined in Sanskrit as *jnana diptir,* or the "lamp of knowledge." The wisdom contained within each of us is a light that dispels the darkness of ignorance, and yoga is the steady cultivation of the right-minded perspective that develops this brilliant inner light. Discriminatory discernment (*viveka khyatir*) goes hand in hand with the lamp of knowledge. When your inner light shines on a situation, it produces clarity, perception, and vision so the true power of drishti is revealed. You will then be able to look at anything and see its ultimate reality. In other words, your power of perception is so awakened and highly developed that you can clearly discern the true from the untrue, the real from the illusory, and the temporal from the eternal.

The Magic of the Breath

Yoga teaches that the fastest way to cross the bridge into more rarefied states of being is through the vehicle of the breath. Drishti or asana alone cannot illuminate the path ahead, so practitioners must also develop specific breathing techniques. In fact, my teacher often said that the whole Ashtanga Yoga practice is merely a breathing practice and the rest is secondary to the breath.

Working with the breath while practicing yoga can sometimes be frustrating. Only a very accomplished practitioner can successfully coordinate complex movements with a calm, controlled breath. When I first started practicing, I was more interested in the end result of the pose than the subtleties of the breath. It took me years to integrate pranayama, or breath control, into my daily ritual. The turning point came when Jois himself taught me the Ashtanga Yoga method of pranayama. After that, I was willing to go to this powerful place within the breath. I have come to understand that without the breath, there is in fact no yoga, and I am now as inspired by the breath as I am by the poses, if not more. Accomplished poses, acrobatic movements, and floating handstands are all just tricks without the steady focus on the breath that is the heart of yoga.

On a metaphysical level, we can think that when we are born, we breathe in, and when we die, we breathe out. The space between these two breaths holds the entirety of our life experience here on earth. In essence, the breath holds our entire life force. Known in Sanskrit as *prana vayu,* there is no direct English translation for this concept. *Prana* means "life energy," and in yoga practice, we are working the winds of our life force when we perform poses and breathing exercises. Even the idea of exercise is inadequate for the deeper definition of pranayama, which seeks to cross the barrier between the physical and the energetic world within. Originally, prana was thought to equate with brahman. The *Yoga Vasishtha* (3.13.31) defines *prana* as the vibratory power that underlies all manifestation. Later, the text distinguishes between this primary life force and the individual life force. Georg Feuerstein states in his translation of the *Yoga Vasishtha* that prana "is both constitutive and operative; that is, it is out of prana that the universe is said to be made, and it is by means of prana's continual flow that the universe is sustained." But perhaps prana is best understood as the underlying matrix that directs the flow of energy and organizes the manifest world.

The *Hatha Yoga Pradipika* describes seventy-two thousand energy channels (*nadis*) in the body and a main central channel called the *sushumna nadi* for the flow of the highest form of life energy. All pranayama practice focuses on getting the prana vayu, or the winds of your life force, consciously flowing through the central column of your body. The full benefit of this occurs when the life energy flows through the central nadi and the light of spiritual awakening dawns within. In essence, the advanced stage of pranayama practice comprises a feeling of timelessness when all focus on the exterior world fades and you enter a transcendental state of ultimate peace.

The magic of working with the breath means that when you control your breath, you have access to all five bodies (*koshas*) — physical, mental, emotional, energetic, and spiritual. Deep breathing is meant to purify the body, release toxins, and stoke the karmic fire within. On a physical level, conscious deep breathing stimulates the cardiovascular system and increases blood flow throughout the body. Exhalation helps remove toxins from the blood through the interface in the lungs, and inhalation floods the blood with highly oxygenated air.

Yoga begins with the humble task of uniting yourself with breathing, pose, and drishti (gaze). In doing so, you unite the five sheaths (*koshas*) of your consciousness in a single purpose. Asana becomes increasingly difficult in an effort to transubstantiate the body into spiritual energy and, at the same time, train the mind to be attuned to higher consciousness. The vital purpose of physical poses is to cleanse the body of obstructions and thereby create a home for the divine.

Relax and Breathe into It

Deep breathing has a direct effect on the nervous system. A long, slow, steady breath is associated with the relaxation response, a specific state of mind and body associated with health and healing that cannot be forced but only stimulated through specific techniques such as deep, diaphragmatic breathing. By inhaling and exhaling deeply, we stimulate the parasympathetic nervous system's ability to calm down.

Breathing is controlled by both conscious and subconscious action, and it therefore gives us access to both sides of our mind. Regulating the breath has an enormous impact on whether we are able to remain calm, healthy, and balanced. The autonomic nervous system controls the mostly subconscious functions of the body, such as heart function, organ function, hormonal balance, immune function, and digestion. The autonomic nervous system comprises two further systems: the sympathetic nervous system and the parasympathetic nervous system. The former is associated with stimulations of stress hormones such as adrenaline and corticosteroids, elevated blood pressure, decreased blood flow to extremities, increased blood sugar levels, and other symptoms of what is commonly known as the fight-or-flight response. The latter is associated with the relaxation response — decreased stress hormones, increased immune function, slower heartbeat, regular blood sugar levels and digestive function, and similar bodily functions. All active practices of yoga use breath regulation to influence the autonomic nervous system and strengthen the neurological pathways that lead toward the relaxation response. Vigorous physical poses followed by a deep period of relaxation increase the mind's (and body's) ability to relax. If you practice yoga, you will regain control over your entire nervous system and thereby also gain control over the total function of your body and mind.

Nasal breathing deepens the state of relaxation, whereas open-mouth breathing sends a signal of distress and panic to the brain. The type of deep breathing taught in Ashtanga Yoga stabilizes the heartbeat during strenuous activity, strengthens the cardiovascular system, triggers the relaxation response, and keeps the mind totally focused within the present moment. Yoga brings you into a deeper relationship with yourself by having you twist your body into uncomfortable positions and then asking you to breathe while you gaze at a single point of attention. The level of complexity

The Five Koshas

According to yoga philosophy, the human body consists of five essential layers, ranging from the outer physical form to the innermost "body of bliss," covering the pure Self (*atman*):

Physical, or food, body = *annamaya kosha*
Energy body = *pranamaya kosha*
Mental body = *manomaya kosha*
Wisdom body = *vijnanamaya kosha*
Bliss body = *anandamaya kosha*
Self = *atman*

necessary at any given moment is enough to stop the mind and create a long pause between the otherwise steady stream of thoughts. The depth of the breath ensures that all of your koshas are fully present and integrated.

Ashtanga Yoga instructs you to equalize the length of the inhalation and the length of the exhalation while practicing to balance both sides of the consciousness. The inhalation correlates with absorbing, receiving, and activity, whereas the exhalation correlates with releasing, giving, and restfulness. For poses that are challenging or painful and require greater flexibility, it may be useful to focus temporarily on the exhalation. For poses that are challenging but require great strength, it can be useful to coordinate the lifting motion with an inhalation in order to maximize the power of the breath. Jois recommended to equalize the length of inhalation and exhalation at all times.

Perhaps the greatest challenge of yoga practice is that you are asked to maintain a calm, steady breath while you move through increasingly difficult levels of asana and coordinate each breath with one movement. The concept of Ashtanga Vinyasa Yoga comes from the notion of coordinating one breath with one movement, which is the definition of *vinyasa*. It is hard to remember to breathe when a pose is so difficult that all you want to do is hold your breath. When things are difficult, fearful, painful, and frustrating, we all have a natural tendency to hold our breath. But if you stop breathing, you stop your life energy. It is important to keep breathing, especially when the poses test your physical and emotional limits. Ashtanga Yoga tells you to breathe, literally, right into the pain, anxiety, sadness, or anything else that comes up. One of the main manifestations of proficiency in a series of poses is not merely the ability to get the form right but the ability to breathe deeply and steadily while holding them. When you learn to breathe freely while attempting difficult asanas, you are also practicing the kind of deep relaxation that will help you in difficult life situations. Sometimes two long, deep breaths can help you avoid escalating an argument with a friend or partner. With yoga practice, you learn to use the breath as a tool to help you face difficulties, both on and off the mat, when they arise.

If you focus solely on attaining the asanas when you practice, you will most likely sacrifice the breath for form, but the ends do not justify the means in yoga. In fact, the means themselves are the ends. Yoga is about the journey and the process, and if there is no space to allow a deep inhalation and exhalation to be your guide, there may never be space for you to be calm in your life. The goal of life is not merely to make it as quickly as possible to the last breath; it is to enjoy the whole glorious ride along the way. If you let go of the need to achieve, you will discover that you already have all the peace you really need inside yourself — between the inhalation and exhalation.

Ujjayi: The Breath of Life

Ashtanga Yoga uses a breathing method based on the Ujjayi Pranayama (Breath of Victory) to ensure that each practitioner realizes the full depth of the practice. We hope to attain victory over the cycle of suffering and past negative behavior patterns. Ujjayi Pranayama is taught in the more advanced stages of Ashtanga Yoga. The breathing done during the asana practice is actually just "deep breathing with sound" and is based on the greater method of breath control. This deep breathing with sound is performed during asana practice in preparation for more advanced forms of breathing practice that are isolated from asana. When deep breathing has stimulated the relaxation response in the nervous system, the breath itself functions as a kind of anesthetic that prevents injury, increases flexibility, and augments strength. Jois always recommended a full ten-second inhalation and exhalation as an end goal to many years of practice.

Each breath has four distinct components: the inhalation, the space between the inhalation and exhalation, the exhalation, and the space between the exhalation and the inhalation. It is important to give a gentle pause between the breaths so you float effortlessly for a moment between each inhalation and exhalation. When you advance to more in-depth breath work that includes holding or retaining the breath, the space between breaths will be crucial. You will notice that the space after the exhalation often induces a slight panic if allowed to become too prolonged, since there is little oxygen left in the body. While it is not easy to face, controlling the breath is meant to stimulate fear — sometimes even the fear of death — so that this too can ultimately be conquered with yoga practice.

To practice Ashtanga Yoga breathing, you must vocalize the breath so that you breathe with sound. Begin by vocalizing the sounds *sa* and *ha* to open your throat. Inhale fully and then exhale while opening your throat to enunciate these sounds. Then close your mouth and allow the power and resonance of the breath to remain throughout your throat, soft palate, chest, and nose. Rather than trying to squeeze the muscles in your throat and vocal chords to create the sound, simply let the power of the breath come from deep within your body. Draw your lower belly in and engage your pelvic floor while you breathe, being careful not to let your abdominal muscles distend while you inhale. You should control full, diaphragmatic breathing from deep within your pelvis. (Chapter 10 explains the *bandhas,* or internal locks, that allow you to steer the movements of the breath with your inner strength.) The rhythm should be slow and steady, so your mind will also be slow and steady. Try not to squeeze your neck muscles, tense your shoulders, or hold your breath. Instead, allow the breath to reflect your true inner strength. Generally, the inhalation is harder to elongate. Try to relax and avoid any gasping for air when practicing.

In addition to all the advantages associated with the relaxation response, a powerful benefit of the Ashtanga Yoga breathing method is the strength and steadiness of mind that you will achieve. Keeping the mind singular in its focus is a great test of concentration. The spiritual side of the method allows you to cross the bridge between the physical and energetic bodies. In a sense, the breath itself holds the key to the moment when the physical transubstantiates and becomes the spiritual. There is a belief that the end result of a successful, lifelong commitment to yoga is the development of a body of light that is as strong as a thunderbolt and as illuminating as the sun, known in Sanskrit as the *divya deha* or *vajra deha*. This body of light is akin to the notion of enlightenment while in physical form. Only with the careful practice of the Ashtanga Yoga breathing method in asana and Ujjayi Pranayama in more subtle practices is the development of the body of light possible. There will be moments during your practice when the world will seem to fade into the distance or into a field of light. Do not fear, just breathe into it, and one day you too will experience the freedom contained within your own skin.

GRANTHIS

The Tristana method of Ashtanga Yoga uses the breath, pose, and gaze to free the body completely so that spiritual energy can flow within. *Granthis* are energetic locks that block the rise of consciousness in the subtle body. The first time I heard about these locks in the energy body, I was not sure what to think. More esoteric than the nadis that correlate with the acupuncture meridians, granthis are hard to understand, and information on them is hard to find. Yoga scholar Georg Feuerstein gives a good list of sources in his *Encyclopedia of Yoga and Tantra,* including the *Chandogya Upanishad* 7.26.2, the *Katha Upanishad* 6.15, and the *Yoga Shika Upanishad* 1.113–4. Even though the ontological truth of the energy body has not yet been verified by Western scientific methods, it is useful to open your mind to the possibility of the experience and see what is "real" for you. Delving into the philosophy that is the foundation of Ashtanga Yoga helps demystify this concept.

The Yoga Sutras describe the mind (*citta*) as being composed of three distinct elements: the ego (*ahamkara*); the mechanical, information-processing aspect of the brain (*manas*); and the higher spiritual consciousness (*buddhi*). As discussed earlier, when habit patterns take root within these three aspects of consciousness, they are known as samskaras. This general term involves multiple dimensions. *Samskara* is the impression or seed; *vasana* is an aggregate of samskaras in active form; and *karmaasaya* is the network of samskaras that forms the subconscious, or the resting place of samskaras in seed form. If the samskaras are in active form, they already control our actions, but if they are in seed form, they are still developing and would be easier to get rid of. These behavioral patterns are so rooted in the being that they run on autopilot and direct our actions without our conscious control. Samskaras can even outlive one incarnation and resurface in a new body in a subsequent life. Negative samskaras create impediments and obstacles to the spiritual path. Positive samskaras create good karma and bear the fruit of realization along the spiritual path. But for ultimate liberation, all samskaras must be released and burned away. While the classical yoga of Patanjali does not mention granthis, my treatment of their interrelationship here aligns with Jois's comingling of the philosophies of the *Hatha Yoga Pradipika* and the Yoga Sutras.

The stated purpose of all Hatha Yoga is to guide dedicated practitioners into a direct experience of the divinity that resides within them. This divinity is transcendent of all aspects of the citta and all samskaras as well. When the prana vayu moves into the central column (sushumna nadi) and rises along the inner planes of the energy body, the sleeping spiritual energy travels all the way to the crown of the head. Along the way, the energy meets negative samskaras that have taken root so deeply that they form a knot along this main highway for spiritual energy. I am intentionally creating a hybridization between the Ashtanga Yoga system outlined in Patanjali's Yoga Sutras and the *Hatha Yoga Pradipika* system as I believe this is what my teacher meant to do. While Hatha Yoga is expressly stated as a ladder to Raja Yoga, there is some debate about whether this Raja Yoga is the Ashtanga Yoga of Patanjali. They could be thought of as different models for understanding the process of enlightenment, and there are many ways that the two systems overlap and support each other. My teacher seems to have had in mind this merger. It becomes difficult to find textual support, and as such, the final interpretation is left open for debate and direct experience.

Like a good plumber, yoga practice tries to remove all obstacles to the free flow of materials in the main line in and out of the body. The granthis are described in the *Hatha Yoga Pradipika* as the three common blockages that most yoga practitioners experience when they begin to feel the rising of spiritual energy through the sushumna nadi. When the physical energy of the muscles, the body, and even the mind begins to cross the bridge into a more rarefied state of consciousness and become spiritual, it is called the rise of the *kundalini shakti*. This energy flows in subtle but strong and palpable undulations along the central column of the body. The literal translation of *kundalini* is "coiled," and this primal energy of the human life force is said to lie coiled at the base of the spine. Usually depicted as three coils, each representing one of the three states of reality (*gunas*), the kundalini is a crucial component of the subtle body. Its awakening is a psychospiritual event that is likened to a direct experience of divinity. Descriptions of this experience range from ecstatic and blissful to painful and traumatic. Perhaps the experience of kundalini is as magical as the divine itself, so all descriptions inevitably fall short of the direct perception.

When the kundalini meets a granthi, the experience is unpleasant and often compared to an intense fire. The full force of the power of the divine within pushes up against a painful obstruction until it breaks through. The three knots are known as *brahma granthi* (at the sacrum), *vishnu granthi* (at the heart), and *rudra granthi* (between the eyebrows). The removal of each of these knots carries a particular life lesson. *Granthi* is also sometimes translated as a "knot of delusion," whose removal reveals the pure, clear light of consciousness. In a sense, granthis are psychospiritual blockages formed by years, perhaps lifetimes, of negative samskaras that must be removed before you can reach various levels of self-realization. Working with the granthis means that you are progressing from the gross, or purely physical, body to the subtle, or energetic, body.

The *Hatha Yoga Pradipika* states that engaging and working with the root of the pelvis while performing asanas and pranayama is the best way to break through the granthis and burn away the negative samskaras. It also says that the root lock described in traditional yoga texts results in the uniting of *apana* with prana in the stomach to produce heat, wake the kundalini, and force its entry into the sushumna nadi. In my experience, the mastery of the pelvic floor on the energetic level helps cuts through brahma granthi and releases the knot located around the sacrum. Some common samskaras stored in the brahma granthi are resistance to strength, change, sexual traumas, trust, and grounding. Working with the interior space of the pelvis helps practitioners gain an access point to the place inside the body where the physical, emotional, energetic, and spiritual all merge. Vishnu granthi is located in the heart center, so to remove this blockage, a deep heart opening must occur. The heart center must be strong and flexible, open to receive as well as able to give. Rudra granthi sits at the center for spiritual energy in between the eyebrows. Its removal is associated with the release of psychic energy and requires a total merging with divinity, supralogical realization, and the surrender of all egoic control. In *Yoga Mala,* Jois states that all the granthis reside in the sacrum, and while this does appear to be a bit of an anomaly in terms of yoga philosophy, it is useful to mention as textual evidence for the granthis.

Working with Ashtanga Yoga to release the granthis also requires the grace of the teacher. Thinking of your accumulated patterns of negative behaviors and memories can be overwhelming. If you try to get rid of them by performing unsupervised, arcane rituals in the privacy of your own home, it will be a fruitless task. Your journey will be easier with the guidance of qualified teachers who have walked the path along the inner body themselves. Being in the presence of someone who has conquered even one of the granthis makes progress along the inner route easier.

Removing the negative karmas that have taken root as latent or active samskaras in the granthis requires effort, patience, and determination. When students confront one of these granthis, the emotional, physical, and spiritual pain can be intense. Without the guidance of a teacher, they run the risk of wavering from the path and quitting when difficulties arise. A teacher can help recast each difficulty into the perspective that all experiences contain the seeds of realization. When the spiritual energy is blocked by one of the granthis, there is often chronic injury that does not respond to traditional treatment, emotional distress that exceeds the real-life circumstance, and a feeling of urgency and breaking. On the other side of this healing crisis is the peaceful resplendence of the free flow of spiritual energy. Without a firm anchor in tradition and the careful guidance of a teacher, students will often lose their way in the dark night of the storm that arises when the granthi knots begin to unravel. Only by exposing the granthis to the powerful light of spiritual awareness, known in the Yoga Sutras as *jnana diptir,* can they be burned away and cleansed. According to Yoga Sutra 2.28, jnana diptir is acquired through practice of the eight limbs of Ashtanga Yoga. Patanjali's main means of restricting and ultimately removing samskaras is through dedicated practice. The *Hatha Yoga Pradipika* equates the citta with prana and the vasanas with respiration. Therefore, by restricting either the vasanas or the breath (according to the *Hatha Yoga Pradipika*) or thought waves (*vrttis,* according to Patanjali), the light of being is revealed. It takes years and perhaps lifetimes of dedicated practice to stay the course and achieve the final result.

Yoga is a timeless tradition whose depth far exceeds the limits of the logical mind. The very practice is based on core concepts that challenge the notions of rational truth. Working with granthis requires a truly transcendental view of life that is attained through self-discipline, practice, and the cultivation of tapas, leading to the dawning of the inner light. Without this, the knots will remain in place, and you will not be open to the true gift of their removal — the peaceful, love-filled state on the other side of each blockage. A free flow of spiritual energy gives the long-term yoga practitioner a luminous body, a clear mind, and an open heart.

THE RITUAL OF VINYASA

The origins of the vinyasa system can be traced all the way back to ancient Vedic rituals that used choreographed movements to consecrate sacred space. By designating the appropriate breaths, movement, and gazing point for each pose, Ashtanga Yoga practice sanctifies the body for the direct experience of divinity. It is not enough to do the poses; the way you enter and exit each pose determines the deeper intention of your personal practice. The practice of Ashtanga Yoga is a ritual designed to erect a temple within the inner space of your body, and on this holy site you experience the magic of personal transformation.

Rather than washing away the sins of the past, the oblation of the asanas is meant to burn away the negative samskaras that are so powerful they wrap their tentacles around you like ropes that tighten when you try to break free. The more passionate you are, the tighter the ropes become, and you feel yourself suffocating under their immense strength. Like boa constrictors, the samskaras go in for the kill when you fight them, gripping your future in death and darkness. The more you struggle, the harder it becomes to get out. Fear, anxiety, and anger only make it worse. In fact, your personal psychological narrative will almost always feed the negative samskaras. They seem to surface when you are least expecting them and usually repeat their destructive pattern just when you think you have moved past them. Herein lies the magic of the vinyasa method: through these techniques, you learn how to surrender, let go, look away, and find a source of light and wisdom to be your guide.

The benefit of spiritual teaching is not always evident in the moment. Sometimes you learn things that seem completely illogical or appear more whimsical than real. Until the moment you find yourself tied in the karmic knots of the past, some spiritual teachings make no sense at all. But when you apply the lessons learned in your personal practice, a simple teaching can feel like a magic spell that sets you free from the bonds of negative samskaras. Instead of fighting the ropes of the past, you just burn through them with the clear light of your own consciousness. This is the blessing of finding the true light of an authentic spiritual lineage. Knowledge and wisdom are so powerful that they can free you from lifetimes of suffering like pure magic. Just as the brightness of the sun is augmented by a mirror, the spiritual teaching is magnified by the power and precision of your presence in daily practice.

The vinyasa method seeks to ritualize your behavior and thereby give you a better chance of recalling spiritual teachings in moments of great turmoil. When you look into the light and ask for guidance in the spiritual path, the answer will certainly come. Your work in that moment is to wait until the answer arrives, even if it takes years or lifetimes. One day it will come, and when it does, it will feel like grace, magic, and freedom. Take time to study and learn the method correctly, because you never know when a certain teaching will present itself as appropriate to a difficult situation. You need to remember everything possible and store it all on the hard drive of your mind, consciousness, and heart. Let the teaching be etched so deeply into your being that it erases some old files completely.

Inside the sacred space of Ashtanga Yoga, you build an altar that worships the highest authority there is — divine, eternal consciousness. Just as the ancient rituals of monks and priests are set by timeless tradition, the movements of this practice are established by its historical roots. Without following the carefully constructed entry into and exit from each pose, you cannot find the temple within. Breath, movement, and gaze are the building blocks of the holy site within the body. Once you arrive at your personal altar, it is time to lay down your arms, surrender your defenses, and open your heart to the power of grace. We all need a resting place from the weapons of destruction we have used on ourselves and others. We need a place to ask for forgiveness not just from others but from the harshest judge we will ever face — ourselves. It is on the inner altar that true salvation lies.

When you look into the light of spiritual awareness, your vision changes, your life paradigm shifts, and your path forever skews in a more peaceful direction. When you gaze back at the net of samskaras that has ensnared you, the power of your vision is like a laser beam that cuts through the ropes of pain and suffering. You win your own freedom with the light of wisdom as it burns away the bondage of suffering and releases you.

3

The Ashtanga Yoga Diet

THE CONNECTION BETWEEN PHYSICAL PRACTICE AND spiritual transformation is one of the most mystical experiences of yoga. It is hard to define exactly how the body, mind, and soul unite in each breath to produce momentous life change, yet practitioners around the world experience it. The high level of difficulty in Ashtanga Yoga, combined with the fast-paced order of the poses, often quiets the mind dramatically. The silent space left in the heart can open the door to major life changes after years of practice. Jois rarely told us outright to change certain things about our lives. Instead, he let the yoga work itself individually for each student and waited for the student to ask him questions. Rather than forcing a rigid or dogmatic approach to the shifts that inevitably come from a yoga-centered lifestyle, Jois allowed students to move at their own pace to total transformation.

Throughout my numerous trips to India, one of the most common questions students had was about was their diet. During the question-and-answer sessions that we called "conference," new students who were feeling the first cleansing effects of yoga practice would ask Jois what they should eat. His answer was always the same: he recommended a simple vegetarian diet. In India, where around 80 percent of the population is vegetarian, yoga students often made the switch easily. Part of the transformative effect of the journey to Mysore for many students comes from the radical shift away from the average American diet to one based almost solely on plant-derived sources.

When I first started practicing Ashtanga Yoga regularly, I too questioned my food intake. The teacher I was studying with at the time never mentioned anything about this. One day, after I had been practicing yoga for about five months, I experienced a particularly healing practice session, and suddenly the foods that I normally liked seemed artificial, unnatural, and unhealthy. I began to question the foundations of my relationship with food. Yoga helped me feel the inner workings of my body, and it became obvious to me that some foods make my body more naturally flexible, open, and calm. My food choices naturally shifted toward these healthier, more balanced options.

Yoga is not just an exercise that demands the right amount of calories; it is a body awareness technique that asks you to feel your body on every possible level. It is the experience of deep communion with the more subtle flow of energy through the body that creates a genuine urge to eat foods that nourish the soul rather than those that harm the body over time. When your daily yoga practice helps you feel the deleterious effects of harmful or unhealthy foods in your own body, you will be motivated to change.

THE HIDDEN POWER OF FOOD

Ashtanga Yoga asks practitioners to go deep within and identify with their eternal, divine nature. Food choices have the power to either assist or hinder this process of self-discovery. Nothing you eat will ever harm the divinity within you, but it may end up limiting your experience of that divinity by blocking energy passages in your physical body. So although food is not who you are at your deepest level, it defines how you approach the world at the physical level. Your food choices are one way that you communicate with the world. Yoga practice encourages a heightened level of consciousness of all the components that go into creating food. Yoga practitioners may come to think of eating as a sacred act of intimacy with the external world and thereby change their entire dietary paradigm.

The balance and joy we find in food are a celebration of existence. There is hidden power in our relationship to food, a latent sociopolitical statement in each tasty morsel that passes your lips. The choices you make about food on any given day are a snapshot into your worldview. Each time you eat, you say yes to a whole way of being, eating, living, and feeling. You also say no to an even wider experience of the world. Eating is an activity that, when properly honored, evolves into a celebration of your highest potential for health and well-being.

The teaching of Ashtanga Yoga is clear about the path to a lasting state of peace being a long, heroic journey that spans the course of many lifetimes. Nothing you can eat will get you there in a flash, but certain food choices can ease the journey. Of course, just because one person prefers to eat apples and another likes steak does not automatically make one or the other a better yogi. Ashtanga Yoga teaches that we are all part of the same world, made of the same inner divine substance, and we all share the same human-angelic heart. Your diet and overall state of health play a crucial part in your choice to live a spiritual life. However, the single most important factor in determining your relationship with the divine is your choice to respect yourself, respect the natural world, and stay in constant contact with the ineffable force that unites all of creation. Whether you eat an apple or a steak is not the bottom line. If you are a mean person who eats a vegetarian diet, practices asana, and lives a life with no regard for the divine, you are not really a yogi in the Ashtanga Yoga tradition. On the other hand, if you are a gentle, forgiving person who practices the full lifelong spiritual path while occasionally eating a steak, you are closer to the heart of the tradition.

Yoga is about developing discriminating wisdom to see reality clearly, so a yoga practitioner must know what food really means in our postmodern, twenty-first-century world. If you practice yoga, you cannot simply turn a blissfully ignorant eye to the farming practices that produce the food you eat. Yoga practitioners are carving out a new niche market of conscious consumerism that affects the world's food production. It is too easy and reductionist to say that because we shop at the organic grocery store and eat at the organic restaurant, we are doing something good for the world. Food choices are also extensions of choices about values, principles, and wisdom.

The bottom line is that, as a yoga practitioner, you are responsible for everything you eat, both on a personal level for what it does to your body and on a local, national, and global level for what it does to society, nature, and culture. Yoga asks you to be really honest about what types of systems you support and to take a conscious stand for what you believe in. As you begin to feel more empathy for the world around you, you have a necessary evolution of consciousness that connects you with all sentient beings. Diet itself becomes part of a peaceful relationship with the world.

AHIMSA: THE YOGIC DIET OF NONVIOLENCE

As mentioned in Chapter 2, one of the most important concepts in the Yoga Sutras is the notion of ahimsa. Literally translated as "nonviolence," this concept forms the first limb of Ashtanga Yoga's eight-limbed path. Within these eight limbs, ahimsa is also the first of the yamas, or social guidelines, for the yoga practitioner's ideal interaction with the world. In Sanskrit, when the letter *a* is placed in front of a word, it radically alters the meaning to the original's exact opposite. *Himsa* means violence or harm, and *ahimsa* means not only nonviolence but also the radical and spontaneously occurring opposite of violence. According to the traditional philosophy, yoga practitioners must uphold the principle of ahimsa every day of their lives. The philosophy also assumes that all sentient beings have a soul and harming another being for any purpose is considered a harmful and violent act. When you apply the concept of ahimsa to the production of food, the choice to be a vegetarian on ethical grounds is easy.

The crucial thing to understand is that the choice to follow a yogic diet is a moral one. This understanding stems from the Yoga Sutras and is embodied in the principle of ahimsa. Far more than merely not harming, ahimsa can be expanded to mean that yoga practitioners must be an active force of healing in the world. Ahimsa is what Patanjali calls a *mahavrtam,* or "great vow," from which no one is excluded, regardless of class, gender, time, or space. This noble proclamation encourages yoga practitioners to take the concept of nonviolence to another level and actually leave the world a better place.

The ethical choice to eat a vegetarian diet is meant to be a reflection of a heart-centered way of living that each yoga practitioner ultimately finds. Ahimsa is only valid as a comprehensive method of interacting with the world around you. It has no effect if you are a violent vegetarian who does harm in the world. Similarly, if you force yourself to eat a strict vegetarian diet, you may be committing a subtle act of violence against yourself. It is not useful to force yourself to be a vegetarian or anything else. Instead, the path of yoga patiently waits for the day when you feel the desire to change your lifestyle into a more peaceful relationship with yourself and your planet. When treating animals as products who are born only to breed and die breaks your heart, then the ethical choice to eat a vegetarian diet is right for you. If you never have that feeling, then yoga still accepts you and gives you space to be who you are.

A heartfelt commitment to refrain from harming others does not mean that we will never have another negative thought. Nor does it truthfully mean that we will never perpetrate another violent act. The timeless vow of ahimsa stems from a basic recognition that we have a choice about how we live our lives. This is the advice Jois consistently gave his students, that is, to eat a simple vegetarian diet and not to harm other beings.

Yoga practitioners are advised to have full awareness of the karmic results of each action. When animals are killed for consumption, the consumer bears the negative karma associated with its death. When you eat an animal, you basically share in the responsibility for its killing. If you love animals, it is only possible to condone heartlessly turning them into food products when you do not view them as sentient beings. Ashtanga Yoga demands that students both intellectualize their connectivity to all life-forms and actually feel it from within. After such a powerful realization, the illusion that animals are not sentient falls away, and the decision to follow ahimsa to its natural conclusion of a vegetarian diet is evident.

"Behind the strength of the body is an energy that is spiritual and keeps us alive. To achieve access to the spirituality, you must first understand the physical. This body is our temple and in this temple is Atman—God."

—Sri K. Pattabhi Jois

Paying Attention to Organic and Local Matters

As is clearly evident by now, the entire process of yoga is about cultivating your own inner awareness, so you need to be conscious of your lifestyle and its impact on the world around you. As a consumer, you choose what you want to support and be a part of by your purchases. Whatever you eat has passed through multiple human hands, sometimes whole countries and socioeconomic systems. If you eat an apple, someone has either picked it or worked a machine that has picked it. If you eat meat, someone has killed or worked a machine that has killed the animal. If you eat butter, a cow has given milk and a person or machine has made the butter. Additionally, there is an entire delivery system that brings the food to stores where you buy it. Every bit of energy and time it takes to produce the food you consume makes a mark on the earth. Each product you buy is a statement about what is valuable to you.

The yoga practice should make your judgment clear so that you can see the path most aligned with ahimsa.

AYURVEDIC GUIDELINES

Jois always taught that yoga leads to self-knowledge, and when students were ready, he recommended that they study Ayurveda, an Indian system of health and healing that shares much with Ashtanga Yoga's philosophy. He also said that Ashtanga Yoga and Ayurveda were "friends." They both date back more than five thousand years. While a full exploration of Ayurveda exceeds the scope and intention of this book, I will share with you a few key points from this system that inform the dietary guidelines of traditional yoga practice.

Ayurveda states that all human beings exist between two powerful forces: the earth below and the cosmic or solar above. Food is a manifestation of the union of these two energies. Foods range on two spectrums: they may be closer to the earth or closer to the sun; and they may be closer to the source or farther away from the source. For example, heavier foods are earthy and include animal products, such as meat and dairy, and root vegetables that grow beneath the earth's surface. Lighter foods like salad greens and vegetables that grow aboveground, fruits, and the juices of these plants are closer to the sun. Such foods reach you mostly unprocessed and retain their solar energy. Similarly, heavily processed products such as canned and frozen foods are far removed from their original source in nature. In the Ayurvedic tradition, foods that have been stored for a long time are considered a source of imbalance due to the length of time since they were removed from their original source.

Some foods establish balance in the body, whereas others instill imbalance. For example, coffee speeds up the brain and often instills imbalance. Similarly, onions and garlic, though they are earthy foods, can sometimes heighten the mind's experience of desire and lust.

The best diet for yoga practitioners is one aimed at spiritual realization; in the Ayurvedic tradition, this is called the sattvic diet. Ayurveda states that the material universe has three qualities called gunas. They are known as *sattva* (purity), *rajas* (passion or change), and *tamas* (darkness or inertia).

Sattvic food is considered the purest and the most suitable one for any serious student of yoga, because it nourishes the body and calms the mind. Such foods are primarily bland, vegetarian products such as grains, fresh fruit and vegetables, organic dairy products, legumes, nuts, seeds, honey, and herbal teas. Rather than being merely vegetarian, truly sattvic food is fresh, organic, or whole. Most important, it is cooked or prepared with love.

The second category, rajas, contains foods that stimulate the body and mind for warfare and desire. These foods were associated with the warrior, ruling, and merchant classes in historic Indian culture. They include hot, bitter, sour, dry, salty, and spicy fare, including caffeine, fish, eggs, salt, and chocolate. Eating quickly is also considered rajastic.

The third category, tamas, includes red meat, poultry, and pork; alcohol; onions and garlic; foods that are fermented, overprocessed, canned, stale, and deep-fried; and rancid oils. Tamasic foods are believed to decrease physical strength, mental awareness, and spiritual focus. Overeating and other eating disorders are considered tamasic behaviors.

It is important to view this dietary philosophy in the context of Indian culture and history. Just as with any new information, you must use your own common sense to see how much of the yogic diet is appropriate for you.

In addition to foods, certain activities and actions trigger the gunas as well. These three manifestations of physical form are constantly fluctuating, and our actions, thoughts, emotions, dietary habits, and consciousness affect the way our bodies feel. Rushing through the day stimulates rajas, procrastination is an effect of tamas, and perfect balance is an expression of sattva.

Yoga practitioners seek to master the inevitable flux of the three gunas, and altering the diet is one of the easiest ways to influence them directly. The Ashtanga Yoga method starts by asking you to begin the process of self-discovery with a careful attention to inner awareness. It is not possible to adopt dietary guidelines from the outside without understanding who you really are inside. Once your self-knowledge is solid, then you can begin to integrate the Ayurvedic diet effectively into your lifestyle. The ability to

The Three Gunas
- *Sattva* (purity)
- *Rajas* (passion)
- *Tamas* (inertia)

control your dietary choices and food intake is also mentioned repeatedly in classical Hatha Yoga texts as a key component of the power of a trained yogi's mind.

CLEANSING AND PURIFICATION

When the body is out of balance for a long time, toxins and undigested material accumulate and clog the system. This often manifests first as sluggish digestion and tightness, stiffness, or weakness in the muscles. After years of consuming unhealthy, unbalanced foods, the body may become ill, and the mind dull and imprecise. Ashtanga Yoga brings the body to a basic level of strength, flexibility, and balance by carefully cleansing all the different systems within the body. However, in some rare instances, additional detoxification may be needed.

Fasting is one of the easiest ways to assist the body's natural purification process. There are many different types of fasts that can help clean different energetic and organ systems. People ideally choose the level of fasting that is most suited to their dietary choices. For example, if you eat a meat-based diet, you should not go totally without food, as that would be an intense shock to your system. Instead, you might try simply abstaining from meat or dairy for one day a week. This day of fasting from one item gives you a new starting point from which to feel your body and may inspire a more permanent shift in your overall diet. After you have attempted a few item-specific fasts and shifted to a mostly plant-based diet, you may be ready to experience a complete cleansing of the digestive system with a full fast. This will help your body clean out long-stored toxins. While there are many beneficial fasts of this type, they are best done under the supervision of a qualified nutritionist. I will share one with you here that is easy to follow.

This plan is for an eight-day cleanse that includes two full days of fasting. Drink as much water and fresh juice as you want throughout the eight days. Abstain from beverages that contain refined sugar, caffeine, and chocolate. On day one, abstain from dairy and any animal-based products. On day two, abstain from grains and eat only vegetables and fruit. On day three, eat only fruit. On days four and five, drink only water, fresh juice, and herbal tea. On day six, eat only fruit; and on day seven, eat only fruit and vegetables. On day eight, you may again eat grains.

When you have completed this cleanse, ask yourself if you want to add dairy and meat-based products back into your diet. If so, proceed with caution and awareness. If you choose to reintroduce these foods, start off with very small amounts and write down their effect on your body. For example, you could note your emotional state, energy level, and overall physical feeling before and after consuming dairy or other animal-based products. Keep a journal both during and after the cleanse and write down the impact that the different foods have on your mind and body. Also take note of how the foods were grown and processed and whether they were created in a peaceful, nonviolent manner.

Yoga practice has many other cleansing techniques, called *kriyas,* which rid the body of accumulated junk and debris. Some highly processed, chemical-laden foods fail to digest properly and can create an immobile sludge that builds up in the intestinal track, decreasing the absorption of beneficial nutrients and slowing the rate of digestion. One kriya (*nauli kriya*) involves isolating and rolling the abdominal muscles in a way that massages the internal organs and intestines; when the intestines are massaged, they become more flexible and are encouraged to release any sedentary matter that has built up. Another technique (*neti kriya*) involves irrigating the nasal passages to flush out mucus and other debris from the sinus cavity. It is helpful for people with chronic mucus-related conditions such as sinusitis, headaches, coughing, congestion, and asthma. Kriya practice is also advisable if you suffer from nasal congestion and consume large amounts of foods that are known to create mucus in the body, such as cold dairy products. Jois only recommended the kriyas to people who were actually sick and suffering from disease, not to those who were merely curious to try them out.

The more closely your dietary choices are aligned with sattvic principles, the less cleansing you will need to do. Almost everyone can benefit from a period of cleansing and fasting. The heightened sensitivity to the inner process of digestion and assimilation aids the development of consciousness that is key to the yoga path.

Practice Yoga, Heal the Planet

While what you put into your body is not all that you are, just as your clothes and your job are not the essential nature of your being, the food you eat is a kind of extension of your being in the world. Food choices reflect the sociopolitical structures you support with your grocery money and create the building blocks of your physical body. When food passes through the permeable membrane of your intestines, your mouth, or your stomach, you become what you eat in a purely physical sense. Although your spirit and being are not composed of this hard, dense physical matter, your body is earthy in origin and heavily influenced by the products you consume. Your spirit is thus manifest in your body and its expression influenced by your food choices via your body.

Although it may not always seem like it, what you say yes to is entirely up to you. You are responsible for all your choices in life, especially your food choices. Only you have the power, moment to moment, to make a balanced lifestyle your highest priority. No habit — food related or otherwise — is more powerful than you are. Food is much more than calories, fats, and proteins. Health is much more than exercise. Happiness is the ever-elusive elixir of life that you have always been chasing, and yoga is the true path toward it. Through your food choices, you can discover exactly how much you value your existence. You will see clearly exactly how much you are willing to allow nourishment, rejuvenation, and celebration into your deepest sense of self. You are a powerful being and a conscious creator in your life. By taking responsibility for your relationship with food, you reclaim a direct experience of your personal power in the present moment.

Do not lose sight of the larger perspective of the yoga lifestyle as you grow more conscious about food. The idea is to live a happier, healthier life and be a better person. The choice to be vegetarian (or not) must fit into a larger understanding of the kind of person you want to be every day of your life. The power of your choice is not about the food. It is about your state of mind and the balance or imbalance of your perspective and approach to life. Your food choices should never leave you feeling alone in the world. There is a way to maintain both your choice to live a spiritual life and yet go home to enjoy holiday dinners at Mom's house — with or without the meat. Living in accordance with ahimsa means you also remove the sense of righteous proclamation from your epicurean dialogue. Ashtanga Yoga aims to teach balance, not division. If there is a voice in your head that separates the world into good and bad based on dietary choices, then the whole healing path of yoga has backfired. If the aim of yoga is to live a balanced, peaceful life, we all need to get over any harsh division we may be creating within ourselves and our lives and learn to get along with everyone around us. Being at the heart of the spiritual world does not mean sitting on your high horse and pontificating to others about what they should or should not be doing. You lose your relationship to others when you judge them for their choices as being different from and less than yours. When you separate your life from theirs, saying that what you do is right and what they do is wrong, you draw harsh lines that are no different from a personal war. Antagonism toward others is not part of living a spiritual life.

Jois's best teaching is the example he lived every moment of his life. The feeling of peace around him was like an aura of kindness and gratitude. It was not food that gave him this aura, though he ate and recommended the vegetarian diet that is almost standard in Indian spiritual families. It was something else that carried through; the food was merely an expression and extension of his peaceful inner world.

In one sense, food can really only nourish you to the extent that you are open to being nourished by it. Health is balance, and yoga teaches the body and mind to regain their natural state of balance. Health is a dynamic equilibrium that holds food, bodily functions, emotions, thoughts, physicality, work, love, relationships, and fun in a teetering sphere. By learning how to keep your mind and body unified in challenging yoga poses, the underlying notion of balance takes root. As you learn to stabilize your poses, you have to learn to approach your body in a new, more balanced way. It is through this new way of moving that life changes begin to happen. When you learn to treat your body differently in yoga, you also hopefully learn to treat it differently outside the yoga room as well. Ashtanga Yoga inspires its practitioners to move out of an unthinking view of food into an enlightened way of eating. But yoga itself is no magic solution. It makes life transformation possible if you are willing to apply the lessons you learn on the mat to every experience throughout the day. Ashtanga Yoga teaches students to understand food from the perspective of creating a yogic lifestyle. If you feel happier eating organic, vegetarian foods as part of your total balanced lifestyle, then the yoga is already working.

The Spiritual Journey of Asana: Yoga beyond Bending

AT FIRST GLANCE, YOGA MAY JUST SEEM LIKE A COOL WAY to bend and twist your body for greater flexibility and fitness. Seeing yoga teachers and long-term students entices many people to practice in hopes of attaining the same sort of toned, slim body. Yet even though some students find their way to yoga because of a focus on the external, the heart of yoga is a sincere spiritual investigation of the inner self. Its highest potential is a constant connection with the highest source of divinity we can know and experience. If practiced with diligence over many years, yoga connects us with an imperturbable, eternally calm place within. But yoga done without the intention of true inner peace uses the body's outward appearance as a goal in itself and has more in common with sports and fitness than with traditional yoga.

While I love sports and fitness and feel that most highly accomplished athletes are deeply spiritual and connected people, I am careful to distinguish yoga from athletics, even though it may ask the body to perform athletic feats. It is tempting to create an exercise routine based on yoga techniques to stretch and strengthen the body. But the deeper benefits of yoga cannot be distilled and separated from the true intention behind it — the goal of inner peace. Toning the body or perfecting a high level of physical performance is never an end in itself. In fact, yoga actually teaches you how to release attachment and identification with your body, as well as with your mind and emotions. It helps you learn how to identify with the seat of the soul within yourself. By challenging and moving past the known limits of the body, you ultimately learn that you are not bound by your physical form. By facing and transcending mental and emotional boundaries — "I can't do this" or "This pose is too difficult" — you get firsthand experience of your limitless potential for greatness. Yoga is a path of liberation from the attachment to both mind and matter. It is a door to the inner world and a life devoted to inner peace.

Physical form and poses, although useful along the way, are not the end goal. It simply does not matter whether your hamstrings are long or your body is toned if you are not a nice person. Alternatively, a person practicing the most basic level of yoga while maintaining a heartfelt devotion to living a more compassionate and peaceful life is perhaps a very accomplished yogi. Whenever excited students would bring in photos of contortionists and other extremely bendy people to show Jois and his grandson, Sharath, Jois would always take time to look deeply at the image. Then his furrowed brow would clear and he would say, "That not yoga. That only bending. Yoga means self-knowledge."

STRETCHING YOUR MIND

Even when students seem to be enamored only with the appearance of a pose, they are often silently expressing a deeper inner longing. Whereas certain cultural systems deem it unacceptable to pursue spiritual studies under an "alternative" religious system, they may permit or even encourage their followers to exercise and to work on getting healthy and feeling better. Thus, yoga is okay because it is a nondenominational, nonreligious system that does promote better health for the body, peace for the mind, and equanimity for the emotions. But beyond this, yoga provides an invaluable tool to help adherents of any and all religions achieve the one lofty aim they have in common: to live life in the light of God, or to know the divinity within on a daily basis. This is the stated goal for all dedicated yoga practitioners, and it is achieved by the scientific, repeated study of the inner self through direct daily experience.

Body and mind are two sides of each human spirit. Yoga practitioners maintain a healthy body in the same way that monks sweep the temple grounds — to provide a clean, clear space for the spirit to live. It is a mistake to think that the goal of yoga asana is only to become strong and flexible. Of course, you will get a strong, flexible body if you practice yoga. But if you focus exclusively on the lithe form you want, you will miss the real gift of yoga: inner peace grounded in perpetual awareness of your true identity as a spiritual being. The physical transformation you attain through yoga is not the result of targeted toning techniques; instead, it occurs when you dissolve and surpass deeply entrenched psychological and emotional patterns; your body changes as your mind evolves.

Naturally, the relationship is reciprocal. Rigidly held dictatorial attitudes, entire belief systems that allow no doubt or modification, prejudices and preconceived notions, resentments, unforgiven injuries and insults, and emotional buttons that lead to explosions when pushed are often asso-

Yoga without a foundation in the philosophy of liberation is just stretching.

ciated with tension, rigidity, and inflexibility in the body. Liberation from these patterns and stresses can be precipitated in several ways: emotional release, acts of forgiveness, intellectual understanding, the deep and restful silence of meditation, or the path of yoga. All of these methods have one requirement in common: courage — because when long-held beliefs start to crack and deep-rooted stresses begin to release, the images and emotions that emerge are often not pretty. R. Sharath Jois said, "A brave person is a yogi who will withdraw all the senses inwardly and try to realize the inner purity. By watching others, we have lost ourselves and lost our inner purity. With yoga practice, you slowly get detached from everything and look inside and try to realize the purest form within."

Yoga asks your mind to be strong, steady, and single-pointed. The intensity of focus demanded by challenging yoga poses tests and trains your mind and your spiritual will. When your mind is strong and clear, you can accomplish any task you set for yourself; whereas if your mind is weak, it will falter and retreat at the first hint of adversity. To walk the complete road to spiritual realization, you need more than just a strong mind. To withstand the test and trials of the soul, you also need a courageous heart.

Often, spiritual practitioners first feel a heart connection with their teacher, someone whose very presence makes them better people. It is said that to be in the presence of a true teacher inspires students to greatness beyond the boundaries of anything they know to be true. When I met Jois, my heart opened, drawing me deeper into the path of yoga and steadying my course in moments of doubt. It is this devotional faith flowing from the heart center that allows you to believe in the practice when things get challenging. The heart steadies the mind and gives meaning to the necessity to remain single-pointed.

Yoga is a path of self-realization that can only be achieved by a unification of body, mind, and soul. The mind lights the path, the body walks each step, and the courageous heart opens all the doors needed to attain the long-lasting result of inner peace. It is the heart that tempers strength with compassion, wisdom with nurturance, and flexibility with balance. Without a strong connection to the heart, the spiritual path remains empty. Our ability to empathize with others, to care for them in times of need, and to be close to our fellow sentient beings exemplifies the best in human nature. The path of yoga is meant to bring us deeper into this tender space within.

WALKING THE SPIRITUAL PATH

A life devoted to spiritual self-inquiry can appear antithetical to everything most of us are taught while growing up. Making the changes that lead to a more balanced lifestyle carries the real risk of alienating those you leave behind. But the path asks you not to make harsh lines of division or pass judgment on others whose path is not yours. Yoga asks you to have the courage to feel your way through to your own dreams while giving others space so that they may find their own dreams.

When you choose for you, you do just that — choose for *you*. But when you try to choose for others, making them walk your path and tow your line, then a small part of you makes them wrong for their difference. Acceptance of all that is means holding everything in a field of love and understanding. Yoga demands that the most dedicated practitioners must eventually have the biggest hearts.

Real yogis love life and are a force of positive change in the world. Leading with their own inspired lives of integrity and intention, true yogis never demand that others follow their path but instead celebrate the wondrous diversity of life. In some sense, all practice is a grand preparation for the moment when you can love every single bit of yourself — faults, insecurities, and all. Yoga works when your heart is strong enough to see the beauty of every crack in the veneer of happiness, to love every imperfection in humanity, and quite literally to hold the whole world's aching sadness in the center of yourself. Somewhere out on the horizon of a life dedicated to yoga practice is a moment of absolute freedom when you see that everything really is okay, no matter how bad it seems, an instant when you unify with the pulse of love as the eternal heartbeat of the universe and an infinity of bliss where you dissolve into presence and peace. Everything up until and maybe even after that moment is, well, just practice.

LIFE LESSONS ON THE YOGA SUPERHIGHWAY

The iconography of the yoga world transports would-be practitioners into an idyllic scene of blooming lotus flowers and gently flowing estuaries. The promise of sincere yoga practice is that this paradisiacal realm of inner peace will one day be attainable for everyone who commits themselves fully. Yet the "real" yoga often feels more like a brutally honest mirror of our life experience than a blissful walk in the park. There is a time when all yoga practitioners confront the injuries, obstacles, and pains that prevent them from experiencing the grace and ease of life on the other side of the looking glass of life. The search for the inner sanctuary is a winding road that passes directly through all the chaos, ungroundedness, past hurt, and trauma that we thought we were putting behind us as we turned toward the serene world of spirituality. But there is no running away. We cannot look for the seemingly impenetrable infinitude outside ourselves; instead, we must look directly within. The only truly lasting flash of effervescence is the landscape of our own soul discovered and experienced firsthand through daily diligence and sincere spiritual practice. The bridge to this highly elusive yet heartbreakingly ordinary world of lasting peace can only be crossed by the most worthy of seekers.

Whereas in "real" life we have work, family, and general activity to distract us from our sleeping demons, in the silence of yoga, we have only ourselves, our breath, and our body to lead us directly into the heart of our own darkness. In the midst of the greatest trials in yoga, we are directed to maintain compassionate disregard of the outcome, observe without judgment the passion play of our lives, and walk the middle way between attachment and aversion. Yoga teaches the life skills needed to attain mastery over the mind, so when you stand at the foot of any seemingly impossible mountain, you will be strong enough to believe you will find the way to reach the summit.

Life is a kind of university where we are each enrolled in various areas of specialization based on our interests and learning needs. Yoga can be understood as the gifted program, because it asks us to go deeper into the core issues at hand. On the yoga mat, lessons are magnified until we find the courageous heart that is able to face them. Yoga is an accelerated vehicle for life learning. When we feel a certain emotion in a challenging pose, it is often a trigger for a repetitive emotional state in our lives. Being on the yoga mat is an emotional isolation that encourages us to take responsibility for our feelings as our own. When there is no one else to blame and the painful emotional cycles of the past reappear with poignancy, the only place left to point the finger is directly at ourselves. It is sometimes easier to befriend the traumas that seem larger than life when they appear in the microcosm of the asana. Instead of reenacting the deeply entrenched behavior cycle of a lifetime, we have a chance at freedom from the past. By focusing on the breath, the pose, and the point of attention within, we are able to stay in the present moment, cultivate a balanced mind, and break away from damaging behaviors.

In the process of accomplishing an "impossible" physical pose, we tap into a part of ourselves that is truly beyond the physical. After we touch that eternal place within, we are more likely to believe in ourselves when we face other seemingly impossible situations. Small moments of personal accomplishment give us empirical proof that we are larger and more powerful than we ever imagined. Yoga gives us the chance to believe in ourselves completely by providing us with a series of difficult movements that we can eventually accomplish with grace and ease.

No matter how advanced you become, there will always be poses and movements that challenge you. When I was learning the Fourth Series in Mysore, I never thought a movement called Parivrttasana A and B (Twisting Round and Round Pose) would be possible for me. This circus-like movement involves a series of headstands, handstands, backbends, twists,

Through yoga, we learn how to live more conscious, enlightened lives by practicing first on the testing ground of our own bodies.

and spinal flexes right in a row, and when I tried it on my own, I always got stuck and could not flow through the series. I remember Sharath telling me to keep walking, keep moving, and before I knew what was going on, my body responded to his teaching and guidance. Even though there were moments when I was not sure which way was up or down, right or left, forward or backward, I kept going, and the pose started happening as though something was being done through me. This impossible movement became possible one day because of the faith I had in my teacher and the Ashtanga Yoga method.

Along the road to realizing impossible poses, yoga teaches us that the real impossibility we strive toward is no mere physical form but a state of inner peace that is completely imperturbable. The consciousness of eternal peace is the classically paradoxical comprehension that the real goal is inherent in the journey itself. To "get" anywhere along the lifelong spiritual path of yoga, we must learn one of the most basic lessons, which is that there is really nowhere to go. This begins the release of attachment and desire that leads to a truly peaceful state of mind.

REVEAL YOUR TRUE SELF

Yoga shows you the way and the spiritual community of friends and teachers illuminate the path, but you must take every step of the journey yourself. Each footstep comes from your own inner fortitude. Each challenging pose that tests your limits is an opportunity to flex your spiritual muscle and develop the gumption to imagine a life beyond what you have known.

All progress along the path comes when you pay the tolls and cross the roads through the ravine of the human soul. You pay with the currency of your body and breath and gain access to boundless energy, true power, and compassionate wisdom. Your story transforms from a tragedy into a hero's journey. Yoga practice has the magic to recast your life in the new light of total presence and thereby set you free from past suffering. In the clear light of self-awareness, you begin to see yourself as the free, happy, and peaceful being you are.

Because you alone do the daily, diligent work of your practice, you will know that you have played a vital role in your own transformation. Teachers, guides, and spiritual friends make the journey possible, but if you do not learn and integrate the lessons, even the best teaching is meaningless. You will look back at the years you spent sweating on your mat and take stock of just how far you have come. This progress will not be measured in asana perfection but in the steady knowingness that you have committed yourself to a more peaceful life. There is perhaps no greater promoter of self-confidence than knowing that you are strong enough to meet whatever challenges you face.

Before I started practicing yoga, I did not believe in myself, and I had no real way to measure success or failure. I judged myself by the external attainment of results and felt frustrated when I could not quickly get what I thought I wanted. After I started my practice, I began to see that I was the master of my own fate and that my thoughts really did create my experience of reality. They defined my daily yoga practice as well as my life. Before I could attain any level of accomplishment, I had to learn how to believe in myself. No amount of effort will produce the desired results without addressing deeply held beliefs about your sense of self-worth. The barrier between you and your dreams is more often your lack of belief in yourself than anything else.

You get what you put into your practice. If you enter the yoga world with a defeatist attitude, you will experience more and more defeat. If you enter with a happy disposition, you will enjoy more happiness. Like a microcosm of life itself, yoga is best understood as a playground where you test out your deeply held thoughts about yourself and see what kind of results you get from thinking the way you do. The belief in yourself that comes with regular practice is more than the self-confidence you get from being able to do certain tasks. Instead, yoga helps you connect with a part of yourself that is beyond the physical, that eternal place where your belief in yourself rests. Only when you touch the stable inner terrain of infinite self-realization do all the poses start to make sense. Once you directly perceive the depth of your own soul through the vehicle of yoga, you truly understand what you have been doing for so many months and years. The spiritual journey of asana finally comes to fruition in your own experience of lasting inner peace.

I always felt that when Jois adjusted my physical alignment and movement, the energy of my being moved in a radically different way. It felt like karmic bonds of the past were being burned away. Sometimes there would be real, measurable physical shifts, and other times there would energetic shifts that I cannot even begin to describe. I have never had an adjustment in backbend like his, and I probably never will again. He would effortlessly take me beyond my mental limit, right to the edge of my physical limit but with no pain or soreness after. Just Jois's presence in the room made all my pain disappear and made everything seem more peaceful and more possible.

If you approach your practice from the perspective of attaining the perfect asana, sooner or later you will fail. Even the strongest and most flexible person will get injured or grow older one day. Eventually, a new generation of stronger, more flexible students comes through. When this happens, it is not time to quit or punish yourself. Moments of perceived failure are often when the most yoga happens. Sometimes we have to gain the perfect yoga body and the perfect yoga poses just to "lose" it to injury or age; thus, we

There is perhaps no greater sense of self-confidence than the certainty that you are strong enough to meet whatever challenges you face.

see that the whole point of the journey has nothing to do with asana after all. Yoga asks you to tap into a place within yourself that has faith in results that are not immediately evident. The only way to rest in the difficulty of the present moment is to have full faith that your ultimate goal, the attainment of inner peace, is achievable. Yoga shows you how to truly believe in yourself.

In yoga, you never "fix" yourself, but you do reveal your true nature. The warm, tender heart of compassion that beats strongly underneath any veneer of cynicism, anger, or fear can never die. In fact, it stays with you beyond your physical form and carries you into the next iteration of your life. The heart of yoga is actually the eternal nature of the human spirit. If you connect to that every day, the journey is already coming to fruition.

COMPLETE HEALING

You may have decided to explore yoga purely for fitness or health reasons, but before long, you may experience the transformative power of this ancient spiritual science working on a deep level of your being. Do not be surprised to find that yoga changes your life in ways far beyond the physical. Ashtanga Yoga approaches the transformation of the human spirit starting with the body and working its way through to the mind and soul.

Everyone comes to yoga from a different place. You may already be involved in one or many paths toward a better life — meditation, vegetarianism, a fitness program, t'ai chi, or chi gong — or you may be choosing yoga as your first adventure in conscious evolution. In any case, entering the world of yoga is an important step toward living a more centered, joyful, and peaceful life. The initiatory phase of the journey is your chance to feel your power as you create your life moment to moment and live your highest potential every day.

Yoga is an open invitation to the spiritual path. It is a path of liberation rather than bondage, a path of direct knowingness rather than rules and edicts. When you start practicing yoga, your body becomes more sensitive and then asks you to live a purer lifestyle. While traditional moral and ethical codes of the yogic lifestyle ask practitioners to be an instrument of kindness, compassion, and healing in the world, the choice to live a peaceful life is meant to be sincere and spontaneous, something that practitioners feel within themselves before acting on it. You change not because your teacher tells you to but because yoga opens the door to a new way of being that you choose to walk through with joy, ease, and grace. The journey into the lotus heart of yoga is a lifelong spiritual practice that bears flowers in this life and beyond. Small treasures abound when you attempt challenging positions that seem impossible but are conquered with time, dedication, and guidance.

It takes a great mind to see unity where there is division. It takes a truly enlightened perspective to see peace where there is war. It takes immeasurable courage to see healing where there is hurt. It takes a noble spirit to see hope where there is despair. And it takes limitless power to see love everywhere around you. Yoga gives you the power to be that force of healing in the world.

PART TWO

Practice

5

Surya Namaskara (Sun Salutation): Where It All Begins

THIS INITIAL SERIES OF POSES KNOWN AS SURYA Namaskara (Sun Salutation) provides an opening into the heart of yoga's physical and spiritual lineage. On a physical level, these movements seek to ignite the inner fire of purification (agni). When agni is kindled, the pose and breath combine to cleanse the body of toxins and the mind of unhealthy thoughts. Only when the inner fire is lit does yoga really work its transformative magic. Performing a series of Surya Namaskara is meant to stimulate the cardiovascular system, warm up the muscles and joints, and direct the mind's focus inward.

There are two variations of the Surya Namaskara in the Ashtanga Yoga tradition: Surya Namaskara A and Surya Namaskara B. The A series is easier than the B series, and when taken together, five rounds of each can be considered a full yoga practice. Traditional Hatha Yoga recommends the practice of Surya Namaskara either before the dawn or as close to sunrise as possible while facing east. Since yoga uses breathing, poses, and gaze to unify and stabilize the body and mind, the best time to perform all asanas is early in the morning before breakfast and the busy hum of life begins. The mind is calmer before daily activities commence, the body is in a residually pure state after the night's sleep, and the air is clean from the trees oxygenating it overnight.

The timing of daily physical practice is also a recognition of the solar-centric universe of India's past. The great sages (*rishis*) in the yoga tradition placed the sun's magnificent presence at the center of their understanding of the cosmos. Every Surya Namaskara is a greeting to the constant solar cycle that gives life to the earth and its inhabitants. However, the symbolism of the Surya element of the practice does not stop at the mere physical manifestation of the sun. It is also a metaphor for the inner light acquired

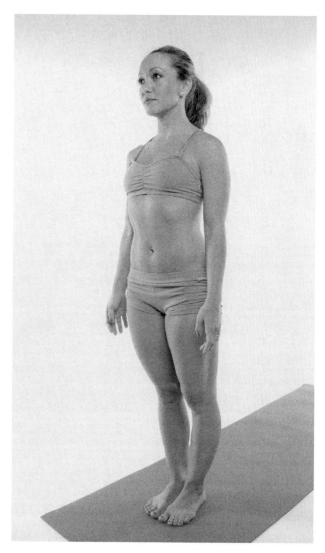

Figure 5.1

by accomplished yoga practitioners. Every Surya Namaskara is a prayer for the practitioner to develop the inner glow of spiritual realization.

While the inner fire of purification creates the perfect groundwork for removing toxins and impurities from the body and mind, this cleansing work is balanced by a sattvic, or peaceful, attitude. Ashtanga Yoga aims to restore health and balance in the body, and the Surya Namaskara requires practitioners to be both strong and flexible. Thus, the solar and lunar aspects of the body and mind become balanced.

SAMASTHITI

Equal Standing Pose

Drishti: Open

This is a standing neutral position that every pose originates from and terminates in when you practice the most traditional full vinyasa method. Sing the opening and closing mantras (see Appendix A) while in Samasthiti with hands in prayer position and eyes closed. Each time you return to Samasthiti you reconnect with the inner work of the practice, regain the composure of your mind, and initiate the next series of movements from a balanced place. While Equal Standing Pose is sometimes called Tadasana in other styles of yoga, in Ashtanga Yoga Tadasana is a different pose that comes in the Fourth Series of Ashtanga Yoga and uses a full external rotation of the hip joints at 180 degrees, like first position in ballet.

Stand at the front of your mat with the base of your big toes and your heels touching (see fig. 5.1). Feel the base of your big toe, the base of your little toe, and your heel pressing naturally into the ground for an even distribution of your weight. Let your kneecaps gently rise and engage the quadriceps while being careful not to hyperextend your knees. Suck in your lower belly and engage the pelvic floor. Let the natural curvature of the spine be expressed without being too rigid. Lift the chest slightly so that the center of the sternum rises and the shoulder blades drop down your back. Let your arms be free and hang in a neutral position next to the body. Allow your neck to naturally lift through the top of the head. Align the central column of your body. Find the perfect mix of strength and relaxation. Do not squeeze or tense your muscles; just be here in a state of open readiness for the practice or pose to begin. If you find yourself tensing your body too much, remember to relax and breathe deeply.

SURYA NAMASKARA A

The student should flow through each of these movements coordinated with the inhalation or exhalation. Only Downward-Facing Dog is held for five breaths.

Sun Salutation A

The flow of the Sun Salutation is fast and requires a high degree of mastery. To help you understand the correct alignment as you flow in and out of the postures, four of the most basic poses are presented here in greater detail. These poses contain the basic anatomical and technical foundation for much more complex asanas. It is important to learn these poses correctly before proceeding to the rest of the Primary Series.

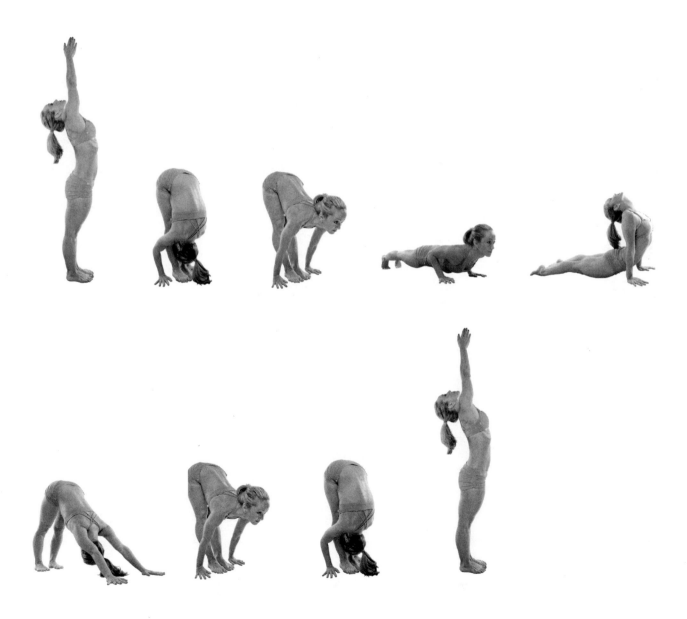

SURYA NAMASKARA B

Flow between all poses as in Surya Namaskara A. Hold the last Downward-Facing Dog pose for five breaths.

Sun Salutation B

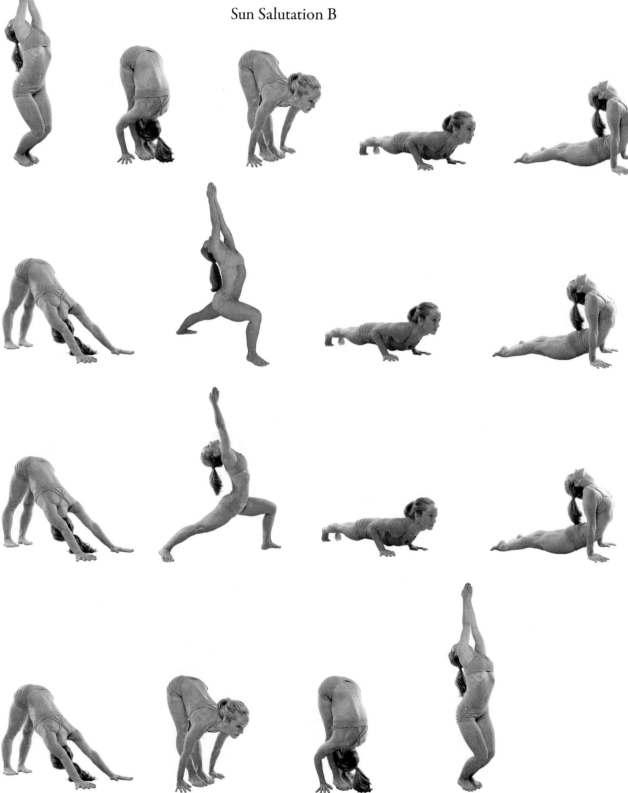

UTTANASANA

Standing Forward Bend

Drishti: Nasagrai (Nose)

Uttanasana is the first standing forward bend of the practice. Traditionally done only as part of Surya Namaskara, this pose sets up the principles of healthy forward bending that are needed throughout the practice. When entering this pose on the Sanskrit count *dwe* as the second breath of a Surya Namaskara A in daily practice, initiate the motion with consciousness and patience.

Stand with your feet together so the bases of your big toes are touching. Lift your sit bones and fold forward while engaging your lower stomach and pelvic floor muscles and elongating your back muscles. Touch your fingers to the floor in line with your toes. Engage the muscles in your legs and elongate your hamstrings while firmly pressing the base of the little toe, the base of the big toe, and the heel of each foot into the ground. Transfer the weight of your body to the center of your feet, testing your ability to balance from within.

BENEFITS

Treats osteoporosis
Stimulates the liver and kidneys
Improves digestion
Strengthens the thighs and ankles
Stretches the hamstrings, calves, and back
Relieves tension and stress
Stimulates circulation

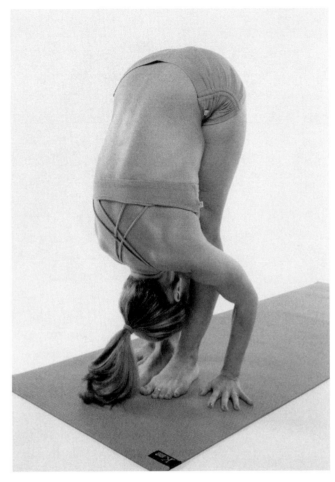

Figure 5.2

CHATURANGA DANDASANA

Four-Limbed Staff Pose

Drishti: Nasagrai (Nose)

Chaturanga Dandasana is a foundational pose for strength and is repeated in both Surya Namaskara and in the movement between the seated poses. The alignment principles established in Chaturanga Dandasana will determine your ability to perform much more challenging arm balances, strength poses, and inversions. Poor alignment will not only prevent

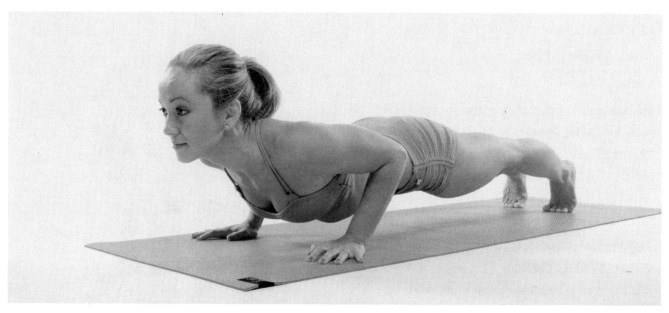

Figure 5.3

you from building the strength you need, but it will also predispose you to injury.

The main structural support for this pose comes from the strength of your shoulder girdle and the underside of your body. Think about the muscles in the front of your body engaging to support your weight, while the muscles in the back of your body engage to help with alignment (see fig. 5.3).

In the Sun Salutation enter this pose by jumping back either directly into it or into Plank Pose (see fig. 5.4) from *trini,* the third breath and movement of the Sun Salutation. If you are jumping directly into the posture, then you should land in the full expression of the movement on an exhalation. If you are jumping back into plank, hold Plank Pose to catch the landing and then lower down as you exhale into the full posture. Your feet should be approximately hip-width apart.

Flex your feet and place your toes directly under your heels; avoid any temptation to lean too far forward on the front of your toes. Engage the muscles in your quadriceps to provide structural support for your lower legs. Draw your stomach in strongly, and engage the muscles of your pelvic floor as actively as possible. Tuck your tailbone under slightly to help your body build a sense of support from underneath. Draw your rib cage inward to help engage the muscles that support your upper torso and shoulder blades, as well as your entire body from underneath. Align your fingertips with the upper part of your sternum and your palms with the lower part. Draw your shoulder blades down your back. The place where your shoulder blade, arm, and collarbone meet is called the acromion process, the bump on the top of your shoulder. This is not a weight-bearing joint, but when it points downward in this pose, it bears weight. Thus, you must keep it pointed directly ahead, your shoulders square and your chest open.

It is crucial that you build strength deep in your upper torso around the latissimus dorsi muscles (in the middle and lower back) and the serratus anterior muscles (around the upper ribs under the arms) to support your shoulder girdle in this pose and avoid injury to your shoulders. Engage your pectoral muscles (those connecting the chest with the shoulder and arm) to create even more stability for your upper body. Finally, allow your deltoid muscles (in the shoulders) to support your shoulders even more. Elongate your neck so your collarbones are open and the center of your chest is slightly forward.

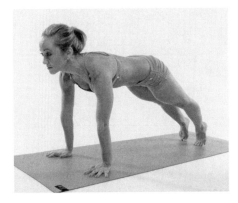

Figure 5.4

If you are a beginner and cannot maintain healthy alignment in the full pose, start off with a simple Plank Pose (see fig. 5.4). Follow the same instructions as for Chaturanga Dandasana but keep your arms straight. You can either enter Urdhva Mukha Svanasana directly from this or attempt the full Chaturanga Dandasana after perfecting your alignment in this preparatory movement.

BENEFITS

Strengthens the arms, wrists, shoulders, abdomen, legs, and whole body
Improves focus and concentration
Stimulates core strength and bandhas
Improves posture
Stimulates the abdominal organs and digestion

URDHVA MUKHA SVANASANA

Upward-Facing Dog Pose

Drishti: Urdhva (Up to the Sky)

Traditionally, you enter this pose from Chaturanga Dandasana and repeat it throughout the practice as part of the vinyasas between poses. Urdhva Mukha Svanasana is the first pose that will help you develop the technique, strength, and alignment that will carry you through backbends. It is critical to understand that this seemingly simple pose is the foundation for your ability to work with your spine in deeper asanas later in the practice. All repetitive poses contain the key elements of a healthy, balanced approach and lay the framework for a lifelong yoga practice. As in all backbends, it is important here to think not about bending your back but about lifting and extending every muscle and joint throughout your entire body to facilitate a backward bend.

Align your shoulders over your palms and keep your feet no wider than hip-width apart. Begin by pressing into the base of the big toe. Think about lengthening through the soles of your feet so your energy extends outward

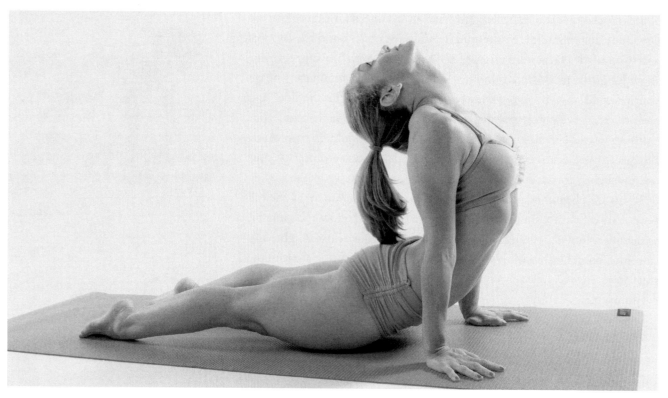

Figure 5.5

and creates length through your lower body. Engage your leg muscles and deepen the extension, reaching through your feet. When your leg muscles are activated in a way that connects them to the flow of energy, your kneecaps will rise naturally, your legs will connect with the pelvic floor, and your thighs and pelvis will lift off the ground. Keep your body lifted away from the ground. Focus your attention on your pelvis; gently push it forward, tilting slightly, but be careful not to flatten your lumbar spine. This movement creates spaciousness along the sacrum and lower back.

Having set up the foundation of the pose in your legs, pull your lower stomach in while activating the muscles of your pelvic floor. Engage your back muscles without shortening your spine, and allow the activation to create space between your vertebrae, lifting and extending your spine up and away from your waist. Stabilize your arms by drawing your shoulder blades down your back. Engage the latissimus dorsi and serratus anterior muscles while thrusting your palms into the mat, planting your knuckles and gripping slightly with your fingertips. As your shoulder blades roll down your back, your sternum will lift; push your chest forward and slightly up to follow this energetic lift. Allow energy to travel out through the top of your head as an extension of your spine and the rest of your body. Be careful not to let your neck collapse while you are looking up. Treat your neck as part of your spine, and allow the lift and extension of the backbend to travel through every joint in your body (see fig. 5.5).

When done correctly, Urdhva Mukha Svanasana helps bring energy up your spine and coaxes it to the spiritual apex of the body and soul in the center of your head. The neuromuscular activation needed to support your body in this pose also creates the structural foundation for more intense backbends later in the practice.

BENEFITS

Strengthens the spine and back muscles
Improves posture
Stretches the chest
Expands the lungs, shoulders, and abdomen
Stimulates the abdominal organs
Improves digestion
Helps ease the symptoms of asthma, sciatica, and fatigue

ADHO MUKHA SVANASANA

Downward-Facing Dog Pose

Drishti: Nabi Chakra (Navel)

Held for five breaths during Surya Namaskara and performed repeatedly throughout the yoga practice, this pose is perhaps the most ubiquitous of all poses. Its prevalence can be attributed to its powerful healing effects on the body. Repeated practice helps students establish healthy shoulder alignment, makes good use of the lower stomach muscles and the elusive bandha area, gently releases the spine in a semi-inversion, and stretches the hamstrings and lower legs.

Enter this pose directly from Upward-Facing Dog. For best results, place your hands about shoulder-width apart and your feet hip-width apart. Draw your shoulder blades down your back and away from each other to create a sense of spaciousness around your neck. Release the trapezius (upper back) muscles. Distribute your weight into your torso so it is supported by the latissimus dorsi and serratus anterior muscles. This helps keep your arms integrated into your torso. Keep your ribs in a neutral position to provide a sense of structural support from the top and bottom of your body; do not squeeze or puff out your rib cage. Draw your lower stomach in and engage the muscles in your pelvic floor.

Practicing deep breathing while keeping this alignment demands that you learn to use your full lung capacity; otherwise, you will merely breathe into your belly and compromise your spine. Release your spine away from your pelvis and feel the sense of elongation between each of the joints. Your hip joints form the fulcrum point for the bend. Deepen the fold at the base

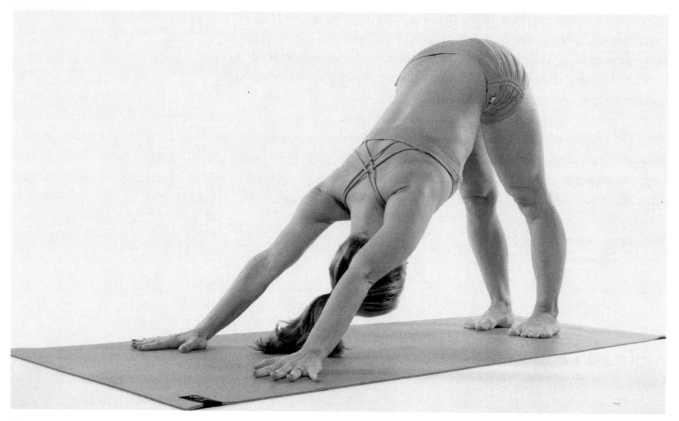

Figure 5.6

of your hip bones to go further into the core of the pose. Lift your sit bones away from your heels and straighten your legs. Press your weight into the floor through your feet between the base of the big toes, the base of the little toes, and the heels. Try to feel the energy flowing from deep within your pelvis through your legs and into the floor by thrusting your feet into the ground and pulling the tops of your thighbones into the pelvis. If all of these movements are integrated, your kneecaps will rise naturally; your legs will straighten further; and your hamstrings, calves, and ankles will stretch. Keep your ankles deeply bent but relaxed. Maintain your tailbone in a neutral position, neither tucked under nor turned up (see fig. 5.6).

BENEFITS

Relieves stress

Tones the abdomen

Improves digestion

Helps relieve symptoms of high blood pressure, asthma, flat feet, and sciatica

Strengthens the arms, hands, shoulders, and legs

Stretches the shoulders, hamstrings, calves, and ankles

6

Standing Poses: Build
Your Foundation

THE STANDING POSES OF THE ASHTANGA YOGA PRIMARY
Series deepen the structural foundation and alignment principles for the
whole practice. These asanas comprise perhaps the most healing group
out of the practice. They are both accessible and beneficial for nearly all
body types, and you can achieve a base level of proficiency in them rather
quickly with regular practice. Consisting of standing forward bends, standing twists, and external and internal hip rotations, these poses provide full-
body stretching and strengthening and can help heal chronic injuries.

The standing poses develop a sense of balance, strengthen the legs and
their connection to the ground, and encourage gentle hip rotation. They
require the body to bend and move in new ways that access the power
points inside the pelvis and thereby help digestion and stimulate the abdominal organs. This relatively easy series of movements lets even total
beginners benefit from yoga's healing approach. Holding these poses for
at least five deep breaths gives the body a chance to recalibrate its neuromuscular awareness. Over time, the standing poses build a healthy and balanced body, cultivate length and openness in the hip joints, elongation in
the neck and spine, and support from the shoulder girdle.

It is essential to be aware of your feet in the standing poses, because they
are your connection to the mat and to the earth underneath. Think of each
foot as being connected to the ground through three main points: the base
of the big toe, the base of the little toe, and the heel. These three points,
when pressed equally into the ground, create a tripod on which you can
stand firm and find balance. The outer edges of the foot should easily remain in contact with the ground when the three main points are pressed
down. Additionally, the arch of the foot lifts naturally when the points
are activated, and the balance occurs with less effort. Be conscious of the

actions connecting your legs with your feet. When you thrust into the base of each big toe, for example, imagine that the energy you are sending out travels all the way down to the center of the earth and then returns to your body in an upward thrust. Allow this upward flow of energy to move from your feet through the interior edge of your quadriceps (front thigh muscles) and all the way into your pelvic floor. In this way, the standing poses create strength, flexibility, and grounding. My husband, Tim Feldmann, deserves credit for sharing the healthy anatomical principles of forward bending explained here.

As you begin working more deeply with the principles of forward bends, you should develop a better understanding of the physical dynamics of a healthy forward bend. Ideally, all forward bends originate deep inside the pelvis — the fulcrum point is the sit bones at the back and the hip joints at the front. The hamstrings lengthen, and the back muscles release to create as flat a bend as possible. The feeling of elongation and spaciousness in the joints is more important than merely touching your head to your legs. To develop your awareness of the depth of forward bends, try to imagine that all the points along the backs of your legs, from your sit bones to your heels, are connected in one long line of energy. Thus, when you lift your sit bones away from your heels, the backs of your legs stretch easily. By planting your heels firmly on the ground, you create a healthy and supportive foundation for bending forward. Draw your lower stomach and pelvic floor inward to create the support and space necessary around your hip joints, sit bones, and pelvic region to encourage a full range of forward motion. This sit-bone-to-heel connection — facilitated by the inner work of the pelvic floor and abdomen — gives you an easy anatomical image to focus on in order to use the body most efficiently in all forward bends.

PADANGUSTHASANA

Big Toe Pose

Drishti: Nasagrai (Nose)

Stand with your feet hip-width apart. Lift your sternum to elongate your spine on an inhalation; this is *ekam,* the first breath of the pose. Continue to lift as you exhale on *dwe,* the second breath, and begin folding forward over your thighs. Draw your stomach in and bend forward from your hip joints to grab your big toes; hold them firmly throughout the pose. This basic forward bend uses gravity to help take you deeper into the pose.

The three points of all forward bends are developed here: elongation in the hamstrings, elongation of the back muscles, and support and release deep inside the pelvis. The fulcrum for the bend occurs deep inside the pelvis at the sit bones. Drawing in your stomach as you bend helps you gain access to the freedom inside of your pelvis and protect your hamstrings from injury. Still holding the pose, lift your sit bones, draw your stomach in deeper, and push your pubic bone back to create a solid foundation from your pelvic floor. Be careful not to overstretch the sit bones and the hamstring attachments.

Now that you have established a sense of your pelvis at the origin of the bend, begin lengthening your hamstrings and release your back muscles. Thrust your feet firmly into the ground, pressing into the tripod foundation (base of the big toe, base of the little toe, and heel) for each foot. Once you feel a firm connection to the ground, allow that sensation to travel through your legs, activating your quadriceps and lifting your kneecaps. Because the quadriceps are antagonistic to the hamstrings (they oppose each other's actions), you will feel a release and lengthening in the backs of your legs as you create stability along the front. Bring your attention to your back muscles and allow gravity to soften, release, and stretch them as you bend lower over your thighs (see fig. 6.1).

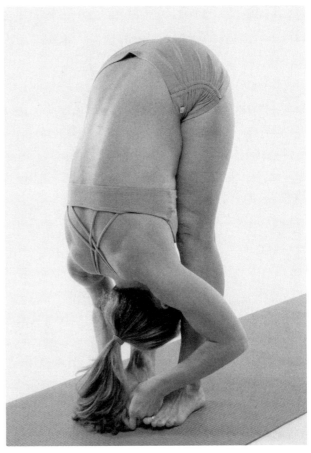

Figure 6.1

Keep your elbows in line with your shoulders and draw your shoulders down your back. Avoid lifting your shoulders above your head and neckline. Ignore the temptation to use your arms to pull yourself deeper into the bend. Instead, allow your breath to create spaciousness in your joints and release into the pose with patience and diligence. If you keep your shoulder blades drawn down your back and let your neck remain free (do not round your shoulders or hunch forward), your spine and hamstrings will eventually release and allow your ribs to make contact with your thighs, deepening your forward bend. Don't expect or try to force your body to achieve this level of flexibility when you first begin your practice. Instead, surrender to a lifelong practice and enjoy the journey.

The leg muscles, particularly the hamstrings, store accumulated toxins in their fibers. If you have experienced repeated bouts of sickness, allergies, or other diseases, your hamstrings may be both tight and painfully sore after yoga practice. As long as the pain occurs deep in the muscle and not at the attachment of the hamstring to the sit bones, proceed with daily practice. However, should a pain arise that is localized at the joint, back off a little and modify the forward bend by rounding your pelvis slightly; if the pain is severe, consider bending your knees until the injury heals.

If you feel pain in the backs of your knees in this pose, be sure you are not hyperextending your knees. Press firmly into the base of your big toe to protect your knees. If you are a total beginner, your legs may even

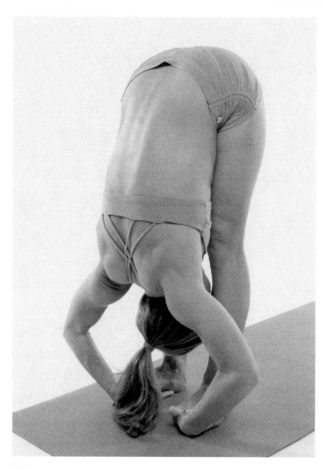

Figure 6.2

shake slightly when holding this posture. Breathe deeply and try to relax. Hold the pose for five breaths and then proceed immediately to the next one.

BENEFITS

Treats osteoporosis
Stimulates the liver and kidneys
Improves digestion
Strengthens the thighs and ankles
Stretches the hamstrings, calves, and back
Relieves tension and stress
Stimulates circulation

PADAHASTASANA

Hands-to-Feet Pose

Drishti: Nasagrai (Nose)

Enter this pose directly from Padangusthasana. Keep your feet hip-width apart. While inhaling and lifting your chest for the first breath of the movement, move both hands as far underneath your feet as possible; allow your toes to reach all the way up to your wrists if you can, and spread your fingers out so you are fully stepping on your hands. Apply the same principles as you did for Padangusthasana, entering the pose on an exhalation, lifting your sit bones to fold forward, lengthening your hamstrings, pulling your shoulder blades down your back, and relaxing your back muscles. If your hamstrings or back muscles are too short at first, you may need to bend your knees in order to place your hands under your feet. If you do, straighten your knees as much as possible throughout the duration of the pose while being consciously aware of supporting your lower back by drawing in your lower abdomen. Once your legs are completely straight, you can deepen the pose by transferring as much of your weight as possible to the front of your feet and pressing into the bases of your big toes (see fig. 6.2). By leaning the weight of your body forward, you simultaneously stretch your wrists, activate your core strength, and develop a heightened sense of balance from your natural center of gravity. Press your feet into your hands and create a solid foundation by using the three points of each foot as though they were flat on the ground. Keep your quadriceps engaged to further release your hamstrings. Keep your neck and arms relaxed as the bend deepens.

This pose prepares your sense of spatial orientation to be more comfortable with inversions. By learning how to transfer the weight of your body from your heels to the front of your feet, you learn how to move your pelvis through space with its own network of support. You may experience some fear at taking your weight forward and further stretching the hamstring, but it is essential to address this fear now in forward bends so that you are ready for it later in more complex poses like headstands. Ignore the temptation to use your arms to pull yourself deeper into the bend. Instead, simply transfer more weight forward into the front of your feet; keep your heels grounded and your sit bones lifted; and allow your back muscles to lengthen gradually. Hold the pose for five breaths. Then inhale, look up, and return to Samasthiti.

BENEFITS

Treats osteoporosis
Stimulates the liver and kidneys
Improves digestion
Strengthens the thighs and ankles
Stretches the hamstrings, calves, and back
Relieves tension and stress
Stimulates circulation

UTTHITA TRIKONASANA/TRIKONASANA A

Extended Triangle Pose

Drishti: Hastagrai (Fingers)

Start from Samasthiti. As you inhale, move your feet approximately three feet apart, rotate your right foot out ninety degrees, and turn your left foot slightly in. To gauge exactly how far apart your feet should be, think about extending them just enough so that when you bend from the waist, the forward foot will be in alignment with your head, thereby making it possible to extend your arms in both directions, while keeping them aligned with your shoulders.

If you are a beginner, align your right heel with the left. If you are advanced, align your right heel with the left arch. Put your arms out to the sides at shoulder height. Start off with the pelvis at the same level and as you exhale, reach the spine out from the right hip joint, away from the pelvis, while rotating outward inside the right hip socket. As you continue to exhale, lengthen your torso, reach out with your right arm, and bend sideways from the hip joint until your right hand makes contact with your right leg. Your left hip will rise and your right hip will drop, moving your tailbone slightly toward your left heel as you reach down and grab your right big toe. If you are advanced or more flexible, you can

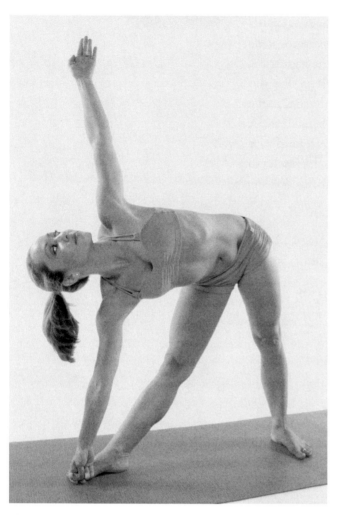

Figure 6.3

grab your toe when you first bend to the right, without putting your hand on your leg.

Hold your toe firmly, pull away from the floor, and engage your shoulder girdle to support your upper back. Draw your shoulder blades down your back and reach toward the ceiling with your left hand. Softly draw your stomach and lower ribs in and engage your pelvic floor to avoid any tendency to overarch your spine. Breathe deeply into your lungs and rib cage, and allow the breath to travel down your spine but not into your belly. Thrust the legs into the ground while spreading your toes wide apart and keeping the outer edges of both feet pressed firmly into the mat. (Engage the tripod — the base of the big toe, the base of the little toe, and the heel — for each foot to keep you connected to the ground.) Focus your gaze on the fingers of your left hand (see fig. 6.3). After at least five long Ujjayi breaths, press firmly into your feet and the earth below, inhale, and rise back up to a neutral position. Exhale as you switch sides and repeat the same motion to the left. Be conscious of engaging the pelvic floor as you come up. Exit the posture with the same level of integrity as you enter it.

Utthita Trikonasana is a fundamental pose that brings the body and mind into balance. It is one that all levels of students can appreciate and benefit from. The sense of connection to the ground that comes from strongly activating your pelvic floor and legs increases feelings of calm. As you develop strength and stability in this pose, your anxiety lessens and your emotional balance is restored. Approach this pose with an open mind, let go of the need to move toward more advanced versions of it, and focus on listening to your breath and body as you enter the pose.

BENEFITS

Improves digestion and stimulates the organs in the abdomen
Increases flexibility in the spine and hip joints
Corrects alignment in the shoulders and neck
Improves circulation
Tones the ligaments in the legs, shoulders, and spine
Strengthens the ankles, core muscles, and legs
Relieves symptoms of stress
Helps relieve symptoms of anxiety, sciatica, neck pain, and flat feet
Eases back pain

Parivrtta Trikonasana/ Trikonasana B

Revolved Triangle Pose

Drishti: Hastagrai (Fingers)

Inhale as you bring your body back to a neutral position after Utthita Trikonasana. Place your feet parallel to each other but keep them the same distance apart. Pivot your feet until the left foot faces the back of your mat and the right foot turns in approximately forty-five degrees. Align the left foot with the right arch, if possible; if not, then align your heels. Facing forward, square your pelvis, hips, and chest; keep your torso aligned with your pubic bone. Exhale for the second breath of the movement as you bend forward from your hip joints, raising both sit bones in unison. Then twist your spine and place your right hand on the floor on the outside of your left foot so your fingertips are in line with your toes. If you are unable to place your hand flat on the floor, you can place your fingertips next to your foot, place your hand on your left shin, or rest your hand on a block placed next to your foot.

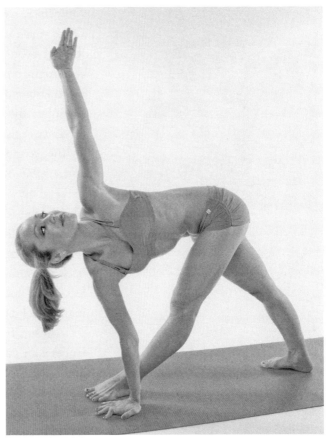

Figure 6.4

Press the heel of your hand, the knuckles, and the fingertips firmly into the floor, as though you are standing on your hand. If you need an additional breath to set up the alignment for the forward bend, make sure you enter the rest of the pose on an exhalation. Once you feel a good connection to the ground through your legs and right hand, twist more from your spine and reach your left arm straight up, keeping it in line with your right arm. Draw your shoulder blades down your back while breathing into your lungs and extending your spine into a full twist. Keep your spine in one long, clean line that flows from your tailbone through every vertebra to the top of your head (see fig. 6.4). Keep your hips level, as though you were making a flat surface with the sacrum (see fig. 6.5). Gaze gently toward your left fingertips. You will feel how your lower body and legs provide a solid foundation and how your upper body and torso lift out of that solid base.

After five breaths, inhale and come up to a neutral position. Repeat the pose on the opposite side. Once you are done on the right side, return to standing at the front of your mat in Samsthiti as you exhale (see fig. 5.1).

The first portion of this pose is a forward bend with the legs in an asymmetrical position. Stabilizing the pose by thrusting down into the three points of each foot helps lift your kneecaps and powerfully activate your legs. Drawing in your abdomen keeps your hip joints spacious and makes

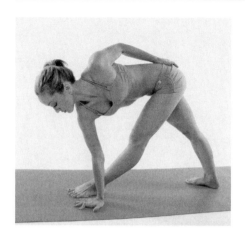

Figure 6.5

room inside your pelvis to bend forward and release the back muscles. Once your forward bend is deep enough, you will gain access to the flexibility of your upper spine, because your supporting hand will lay flat on the ground and provide the foundation for a healthy twist. When you have a good sense of the control in your pelvis, you will be able to stabilize your hip joints and fold from deep within without compromising the structural integrity of the pose.

The second portion of this pose is a twist that extends throughout your entire spine. All twisting motions are supported by the elongation of the postural muscles in your back, neck, and spine. Drawing your stomach and rib cage in is crucial, so you can provide the structural support needed for spinal flexibility. Create space between each joint of your spine by breathing fully and elongating rather than crunching the joints. To support your upper back and stimulate the muscles that facilitate bending the upper spine, you must keep your shoulder blades down your back, and your neck must remain free. Press equally into both legs and feet to stabilize your pelvis.

Parivrtta Trikonasana sometimes brings up issues of fear, because it challenges your sense of balance. Many practitioners get frustrated when their hands do not touch the floor on the first try. Using your breath to deepen and release your hamstrings and spine on every exhalation will allow you to go deeper. The breath is the key to calming your nervous system and gaining mastery over your mind and body.

BENEFITS

Cleanses the internal organs
Helps relieve symptoms of asthma
Stimulates digestion
Opens the chest and improves breathing
Strengthens the lower back, spine, shoulders, legs, and groin
Stretches the hamstrings, spine, hips, upper back, and chest
Improves sense of balance

UTTHITA PARSVAKONASANA/ PARSVAKONASANA A

Extended Side Angle Pose

Drishti: Hastagrai (Fingers)

From Samsthiti, inhale as you step out to a relatively wide stance ranging from three-and-a-half to four feet, depending on your height and body proportions. Stretch your arms out to the sides while rotating your right foot out ninety degrees and aligning the right heel with the left arch. As you exhale, press your legs firmly into the ground and bend your right knee until it is directly over your right ankle, your right thigh is parallel to the ground, and your right shin is perpendicular to the ground.

Sink from deep inside your right hip joint and release your torso toward the floor on the right side while lowering your right hand to the ground. Press your right knee into your right arm, extend your left arm over your head, draw your shoulder blades down your back, and gaze up at your left fingertips. If you are not able to reach the floor comfortably with your right hand, hook your right forearm on your right thigh and press down firmly while releasing your right hip joint as much as possible. Stay in this position for five breaths and then see if you can reach the floor with your right fingertips or possibly place your palm flat on the floor.

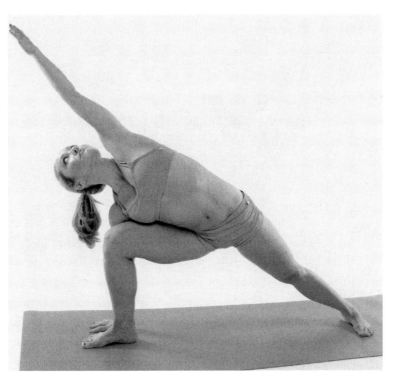

Figure 6.6

Thrust your legs firmly into the ground as your support and connection to the earth. This should lift your left kneecap. Be careful not to sink too low in your hip joints, allow your knee to move past your toes, lose the sense of strength in your legs, or collapse into your left knee. Advanced practitioners can shift their knee to the center of the foot.

Hold the pose, reaching your left hip, rib cage, and armpit toward the ceiling, while folding and releasing from deep inside your right hip joint and strengthening your right shoulder. Draw your abdomen in and feel your pelvic floor lifting. Ignore the temptation to overarch your back or turn your left hip forward to compensate for a lack of flexibility.

Draw your shoulder blades down your back, creating spaciousness around your neck and opening the area around your sternum. Elongate your spine while keeping your neck in line, and reach out through your whole spine. After at least five deep breaths, push into your legs and inhale as you return to standing position with your feet wide apart and parallel. On an exhalation, repeat the pose on the opposite side.

BENEFITS

Strengthens the legs, back, abdomen, shoulders, groin, ankles, and feet
Relieves backache
Treats constipation
Cleanses abdominal organs
Increases stamina
Lessens menstrual discomfort

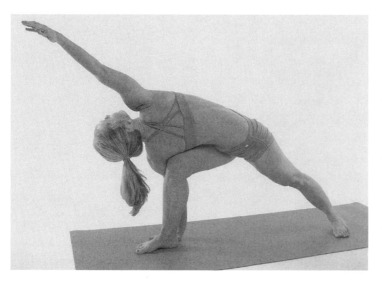

Figure 6.7

PARIVRTTA PARSVAKONASANA/ PARSVAKONASANA B

Revolved Side Angle Pose

Drishti: Hastagrai (Fingers)

Enter this pose directly from Utthita Parsva-konasana. Keep your stance relatively wide, with your feet three-and-a-half to four feet apart, depending on your height and body proportions. Inhale as you stretch your arms out to the sides parallel with the floor, rotate your right foot out ninety degrees, rotate your left foot a few degrees in the direction of your right foot, and align your left heel with the right arch. If you are attempting this pose for the first time, exhale as you come down onto your left knee while pivoting on the ball of your left foot (see fig. 6.8; please note that the pose in this figure is facing the left side to better illustrate the connection between the torso, bent knee, bound arm, and hand placement). Turn your torso forward to face your right leg. Bend your right knee until it is over your right ankle and your right thigh is parallel to the ground.

Clasp your right knee with your right hand and pull it toward the center of your torso, rotating it slightly inward from the hip joint. Exhale and suck in your stomach (but keep it soft); reach your left arm as far around your right knee as possible, leading with your elbow. Once your upper left arm is hooked around your right knee, press your left hand — fingertips and palm — firmly into the ground.

Once you are stable in this position, place your right hand on your sacrum and straighten your left leg on an inhalation. Find your balance and reach your right arm over your head, forming an extension of the long line of your body; gaze up at your fingertips. Keep thrusting your right knee forward to maintain contact with your upper right arm (see fig. 6.9). If you are still comfortable in the pose and your upper left arm is still in contact with your right knee, push your left heel down toward the ground, rotating your left thigh outward to enter the pose fully (see fig. 6.7).

Ignore the temptation to let go of the depth of the bend in your right knee and the spinal twist when you straighten your left leg and place your left heel on the ground. Remember that this is a twisting pose above all else. Draw your shoulder blades down your back while extending through each vertebra in your spine. See if you can twist a little more on every exhalation by drawing your lower ribs in and breathing into your full lung capacity. After you have performed five breaths in the full pose, inhale and return to a neutral, wide-legged position. Exit the pose the same way you entered. Exhale and repeat the pose to the opposite side, then return to Samsthiti.

Advanced practitioners should attempt to enter the pose without going down onto their knees first; simply move directly into the twist with both heels fully planted on the ground. This is the first pose where you begin to work on the sense of "binding" in a twisting position. By locking your upper arm around your bent knee, you develop the release in your shoulder and hip joints that facilitates deeper twists like Marichasana C and D. If you have a hard time with this pose, take extra breaths at each stage to deepen your ability to twist.

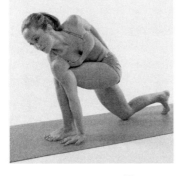

Figure 6.8

BENEFITS

Strengthens the legs, back, abdomen, groin, ankles, and feet
Relieves backache and sciatica
Treats constipation
Cleanses abdominal organs
Stretches the hip flexors, shoulders, and spine
Improves digestion and elimination
Helps sense of balance

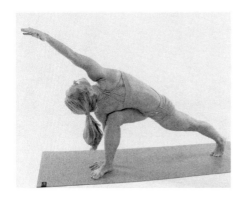

Figure 6.9

PRASARITA PADOTTANASANA A

Wide-Legged Forward Bend A

Drishti: Nasagrai (Nose)

Standing at the front of your mat in Samasthiti, inhale as you step out to the right and place your feet between three and four feet apart, depending on your height (shorter people should take a narrower stance, and taller people should take a wider stance). Keep your feet parallel to each other and align your heels. Stretch your arms out to the sides. Place your hands on your waist to set up for the movement. Establish the alignment of the forward bend by pressing your feet firmly into the floor at the three main points and engaging your legs. With your hands on your waist, lift your spine, feeling your life energy extending out through the top of your head; do not overextend your back. Exhale and lift your sit bones away from your heels as you bend forward from deep inside your hip joints. Place your hands firmly on the floor at least in line with toes. Beginners can widen their stance if necessary to achieve this placement. Release your back muscles, lengthen your hamstrings and all the muscles in the backs of your legs, stabilize the front of each leg, softly draw your abdomen in, and lift your pelvic floor. Inhale again as you look up so as to reach the spine upward, creating even more space in the spine. Finally, exhale and enter the pose completely, placing the top of your head on the floor while keeping your shoulder blades down your back. It is crucial that you coordinate the

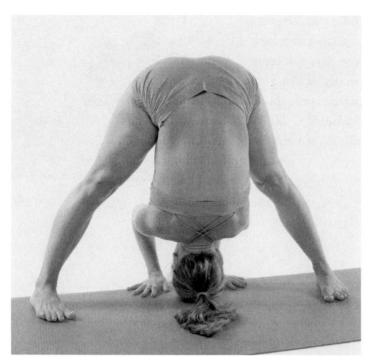

Figure 6.10

downward motions with exhalations and upward motions with inhalations so that you control your sense of balance and do not get dizzy.

All steps leading up to the full asana (see fig. 6.10) are meant to establish the alignment principles of the pose. Remember to work with the three main points of forward bending: lengthening the back, stretching the whole back of each leg, and drawing in the abdomen for structural support. Maintain a healthy sense of alignment in the pose, keep your legs actively thrusting into the floor, and draw your shoulder blades down your back. Allow your weight to travel gently to the top of your head as you shift your pelvis forward as though you were moving toward a headstand. Soften your hip flexors and hip joints so you can slide your torso between your thighs. To deepen the forward bend, draw your energy up along the inner length of your thighs. Feel a connection between the bases of your big toes, the inside of your quadriceps, and your pelvic floor. The more you work this inner energy line, the easier it will be to release the hip flexors and other exterior muscles around your hips that can make forward bends uncomfortable.

Advanced practitioners may find it necessary to shift their hands farther back between their feet so the fingertips are in line with the heels rather than the toes. Finding the three points of healthy forward bends in Prasarita Padottanasana A prepares you for deeper wide-legged forward bends, such as Upavistha Konasana, Supta Konasana, and Kurmasana. By releasing your hip joints enough to allow your torso to slide between your thighs, you are also beginning to prepare for more advanced leg-behind-the-head poses, like Supta Kurmasana.

For beginners, this is often a more approachable forward bend than Padangusthasana or Padahastasana, because you can widen your legs enough to move your head close to the floor. This pose is also a good substitute for Padangusthasana or Padahastasana during pregnancy.

Take five breaths in full pose, then inhale and look up while keeping your hands on the floor. Exhale as you settle your weight into your hip joints, and inhale as you return to a neutral upright position, bringing your hands to your waist as you come up.

Benefits

Treats headache, fatigue, and depression
Stimulates the brain, liver, and kidneys
Improves digestion

Strengthens the back, inner thighs, and ankles
Stretches the hamstrings, calves, and back
Relieves tension and stress
Stimulates circulation
Tones the abdominal organs and muscles

Prasarita Padottanasana B

Wide-Legged Forward Bend B

Drishti: Nasagrai (Nose)

In the Ashtanga Yoga sequence, the four Prasarita Padottanasana poses follow each other directly. After completing A, keep your feet and legs in the same position, and
then inhale as you stretch your arms out to the sides for
the first breath of B. Establish the alignment of the forward bend by pressing firmly into the floor, ground all
three main points of each foot, engage your legs, and look straight ahead.
Exhale as you place your hands on your hips. Look up and inhale again,
creating length in your spine, then exhale as you fold forward from deep
within your pelvis; keep your hands firmly grasping your hips, and lift your
sit bones away from your heels. Release your back muscles, lengthen your
hamstrings and all the muscles in the backs of your legs, stabilize the front
of each leg, softly draw your abdomen in, and lift your pelvic floor (see
fig. 6.11). As you fold more deeply forward, the hands will slide toward the
back of the pelvis to facilitate deep forward bending.

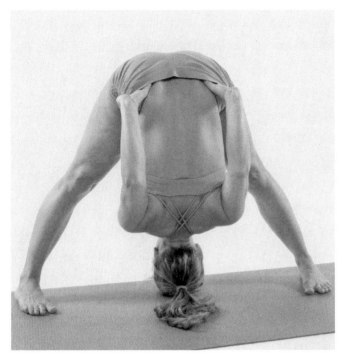

Figure 6.11

Since your hands remain on your hips rather than on the ground, this
pose challenges your sense of balance. Many practitioners feel as though
they are going to fall forward and therefore do not experience their true
range of flexibility. Ideally, your head is in the same position as in all other
Prasarita poses, just without the support of your hands. You challenge
your sense of balance and spatial orientation by asking your pelvis to support itself while shifting your weight forward. Establishing a healthy sense
of balance in B allows you to build the kind of core strength and awareness of the back that facilitates easy inversions and stamina later in the
practice.

Remain in the pose for five breaths, then inhale as you come up, keeping
your hands on your hips, and exhale once you return to an upright position.

Benefits

Treats headache, fatigue, and depression
Stimulates the brain, liver, and kidneys

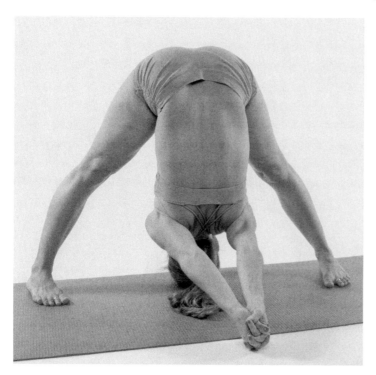

Figure 6.12

Improves digestion

Strengthens the back, inner thighs, and ankles

Stretches the hamstrings, calves, and back

Relieves tension and stress

Stimulates circulation

Tones the abdominal organs and muscles

Increases sense of balance

PRASARITA PADOTTANASANA C

Wide-Legged Forward Bend C

Drishti: Nasagrai (Nose)

After completing Prasarita Padottanasana B, keep your feet in the same position and inhale as you lift your arms out to the sides. Deepen the alignment principles of the forward bend and exhale as you interlock your fingers with palms facing each other behind your back (near your sacrum). Keep your fingers laced, inhale, and look and reach upward without over-arching your back. Exhale, lift your sit bones away from your heels, and fold forward to place your head firmly on the floor; reach your hands toward the floor over the top of your head. You may find it useful to let your back round slightly to get your head to the floor, but eventually you will be able to do this with a straight spine (see fig. 6.12).

Lean your weight forward to the front of your feet and allow gravity to help your shoulders open. Ignore the temptation to overengage and pinch your shoulder blades together. Instead, let them release and travel down your back. A good tip for beginners is either to release your neck toward the floor (if your head isn't touching the mat) or to round your neck so your head will reach the floor more comfortably. This keeps your neck long and free while facilitating a healthy opening of the shoulders.

Prasarita Padottanasana C is crucial for every practitioner of Ashtanga Yoga, because it creates the openness in the shoulders that almost all seated poses demand. If you cannot release your shoulders with the aid of gravity, you will find it even harder to do so while seated. Stretching your shoulders over the top of your head toward the floor teaches your body the same rotation necessary in the Marichasana and Kurmasana sequences.

After five breaths in this pose, you might like to try the complete, advanced version (see fig. 6.13). Stay in your forward bend and keep your fingers laced. Bend your elbows, rotate your shoulder joints forward, flip your hands outward, and straighten your arms again. It should feel slightly uncomfortable. Be more conscious of rotating your shoulder joints than of pushing your arms to the ground. Take another five breaths. When you get proficient at this movement, you can move directly into the more advanced version and skip the easier option. Inhale as you return to standing, by shifting your weight toward your heels. Then exhale and place your hands on your waist.

BENEFITS

Treats headache, fatigue, and depression
Stimulates the brain, liver, and kidneys
Improves digestion
Strengthens the back, inner thighs, and ankles
Stretches the shoulders, hamstrings, calves, and
    back
Relieves tension and stress
Stimulates circulation
Tones the abdominal organs and muscles
Increases sense of balance

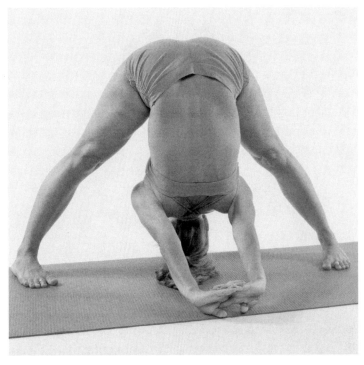

Figure 6.13

PRASARITA PADOTTANASANA D

Wide-Legged Forward Bend D

Drishti: Nasagrai (Nose)

After exiting Prasarita Padottanasana C, keep your hands on your waist. Begin D by inhaling, gazing up and lifting your spine and feeling your life energy extending out through the top of your head; do not arch your back. Press firmly into the floor, grounding all three main points of each foot and engage your legs. Exhale as you lift your sit bones away from your heels to fold forward from deep within your pelvis; grab your big toes with your thumbs, index fingers, and middle fingers. Release your back muscles, lengthen your hamstrings and all the muscles in the backs of your legs, stabilize the front of each leg, softly draw your abdomen in, and lift your pelvic floor. Inhale again, look up, lift your head, stretch and lengthen your spine, and finally exhale as you enter the complete pose, placing the top of your head on the floor. Hold the pose while you take five breaths.

Draw your shoulder blades down your back, align your elbows with your wrists, and your head with your arches. If you are unable to touch

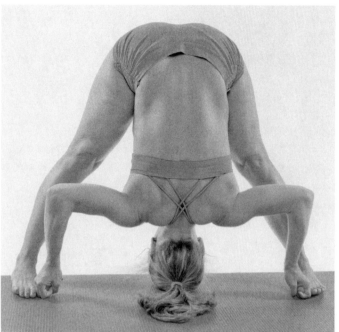

Figure 6.14

your head to the floor, simply let gravity elongate your hamstrings and back muscles while you breathe deeply. Press firmly into your feet and allow the strength of your legs to be your sense of support. Engage your arms just enough to provide support for your shoulder blades but soft enough to allow your neck to remain free (see fig. 6.14). Be careful not to press your big toes into the mat but, just as in Trikonasana A, pull lightly with your hands away from the floor. Remember that the strength, stability, and opening of the forward bend happen from within the pelvis, not from the arms. This pose allows you to combine the supported feeling from A with the unsupported feeling from B. The release of your hip joints and hamstrings, combined with the inner lift of your abdomen integrates strength and flexibility.

Exit the pose by inhaling and looking up while still holding on to your toes. Exhale as you settle your weight into your hip joints. Inhale as you return to an upright position bringing your hands up along the way; exhale and return to Samsthiti.

Benefits

Treats headache, fatigue, and depression
Stimulates the brain, liver, and kidneys
Improves digestion
Strengthens the back, inner thighs, and ankles
Stretches the hamstrings, calves, and back
Relieves tension and stress
Stimulates circulation
Tones the abdominal organs and muscles

Parsvottanasana

Intense Side Stretch Pose

Drishti: Padhayoragai (Toes)

Starting in Samasthiti at the front of your mat, grab your elbows behind your back. If this is easy for you, then press your fingertips together at your lower back until your hands find their way into prayer position behind your back. Press the outer edges of your hands into your spine and gently arch your back to make space for your hands. Inhale as you step out to the right, pivoting your right foot until it faces the back of your mat. Rotate your left foot inward between forty-five and sixty degrees. Align your right heel with the left arch, and square your pelvis toward the back of your mat, to the right in line with your foot. Exhale as you bend from your sit bones and reach forward with your chest, elongating your back and hamstrings while stabilizing your weight in your pelvis to enter the pose (see fig. 6.15).

Draw your abdomen in and lift your sit bones as you fold forward; firmly press your legs into the floor. Remember to ground all three main points of each foot as you reach into the pose. Keep your pelvis and sacrum as level as possible and avoid twisting to one side to enter the posture. As you bend, think about rotating your right thigh slightly inward, pulling up energetically along the inside of your right leg from the base of your big toe through the inner side of your quadriceps and all the way

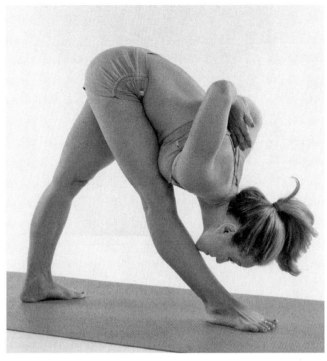

Figure 6.15

into your pelvic floor. Keep your sternum in line with your pubic bone and right knee. Lift your elbows and press the heels of your hands together firmly to deepen the stretch in your shoulders and keep your chest open (see fig. 6.16).

The slight inward rotation of your right leg allows you to deepen the fold between your hips, your torso, and the floor. This same precision is needed in twists, and although this pose is not a twist, it provides a safe, easy way to work on the flexibility you need at the base of your pelvis for deep twisting. Similarly, pressing your hands together rotates your shoulders and prepares you for the movement necessary in the seated poses.

If you are more advanced, Parsvottanasana can even improve your ability to lift up into arm balances by allowing a deeper dorsi flexion of the wrists. After five breaths on the right side, come up on an inhalation while engaging the pelvic floor. Pivot your feet, and repeat the pose to the left for five breaths. Inhale as you come up, and return to Samsthiti.

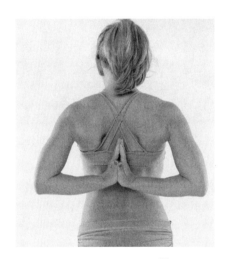

Figure 6.16

BENEFITS

Strengthens the legs, spine, and hips
Stretches the hamstrings, shoulders, and wrists
Helps relieve symptoms of flat feet
Improves digestion
Teaches balance
Stimulates the abdominal organs
Calms the brain

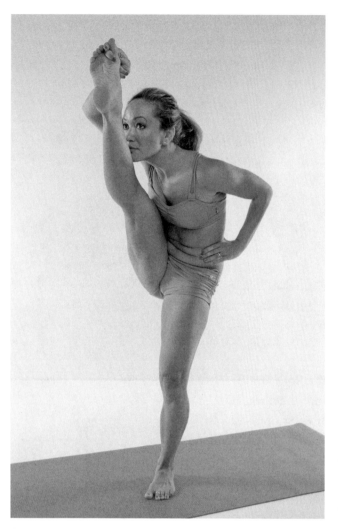

Figure 6.17

UTTHITA HASTA PADANGUSTHASANA A, B, AND C

Extended Hand-to-Big-Toe Pose

Drishti A: Padhayoragrai (Toes)

Drishti B: Parsva (Side)

Drishti C: Padhayoragrai (Toes)

This dynamic series of three linked poses marks the official beginning of the Ashtanga Yoga Primary Series. I have included it with the standing poses because Utthita Hasta Padangusthasana and those that immediately follow are performed from a standing position, so the technical and anatomical information from the previous poses applies here as well. Utthita Hasta Padangusthasana is best understood as a balancing pose rather than a stretching pose. Maintaining a healthy sense of balance in both the body and the mind is the key to performing this pose well.

Standing in Samasthiti, pick a spot anywhere in front of you on which to focus. The smaller your point of focus, the easier it will be to maintain your balance. Having established your point of attention, transfer the weight of your body onto your left leg and allow your right foot to rise naturally off the ground. Stabilize your hip joints and pelvis, and keep both sit bones at the same height. Inhale as you lift your right leg, initiating the motion from deep within the center of your body, and grab hold of your big toe with the first three fingers of your right hand. Engage the quadriceps of both legs by thrusting into the ground through your left leg and reaching forward and away from your body with your right. Lift your leg only as high as your hamstring flexibility permits, and do not try to get it higher by lifting your hips or destabilizing your pelvis. As you clasp your toe firmly with your fingers, you may find that thrusting your toe into your hand helps straighten your right knee.

Draw your stomach in, engage your pelvic floor, and exhale as you elongate your spine and fold forward toward your right leg. Wait until you feel a solid sense of balance and have relatively open hamstrings before you try to fold forward too deeply. If you can balance but lack flexibility, fold forward as much as possible, initiating the forward bend from deep within your pelvis. If you are advanced, touch your chin to your right shin and switch your gaze to the toes of your right foot. Advanced practitioners are able to move directly into this gaze from the moment they assume the pose (see fig. 6.17).

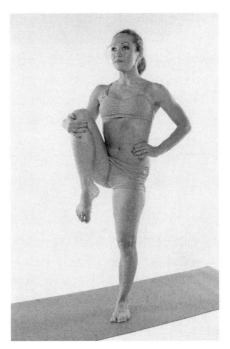

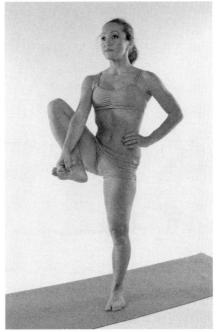

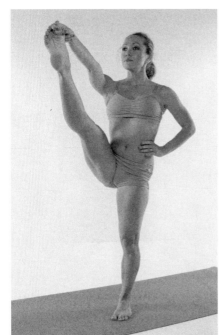

Figure 6.18   *Figure 6.19*   *Figure 6.20*

Beginners will find the full version of the pose challenging. If you cannot hold your toe, hold either your knee or your big toe with your leg bent (see figs. 6.18 and 6.19). If you can balance while holding your right toe with a bent leg, try to straighten your leg as much as possible but don't bend forward until you can balance there (see fig. 6.20).

Hold each pose in this sequence for five breaths. Move directly from Utthita Hasta Padangusthasana A into B; continue at the same level, either a beginner with the modification or an advanced practitioner with the full pose. Before beginning to move your right leg to the side, turn your head and find a new spot out to the left for your eyes to focus on. Exhale as you bring your right leg out to the side (see fig. 6.21). Contract the muscles of your pelvic floor to create a solid foundation in the root of your pelvis, then rotate your hip joint externally to bring your leg out to the side on an exhalation. Often the leg that is out to the side wants to bring the hip with it on its journey, so resist the urge to lift one hip higher than the other. The purpose of this pose is not to rotate your pelvis but to rotate your hip joint while maintaining stability in your pelvis. It is therefore essential that the movement that takes your leg out to the side comes from a deep rotation of the hip joint without compromising the structural integrity of the pelvis. To go deeper, drop your right greater trochanter (near the top of the thighbone) and move the head of the femur (thighbone) inside the hip socket. This will create even more outward rotation and eventually lift the right leg higher. But remember that the purpose of the pose is to find stability.

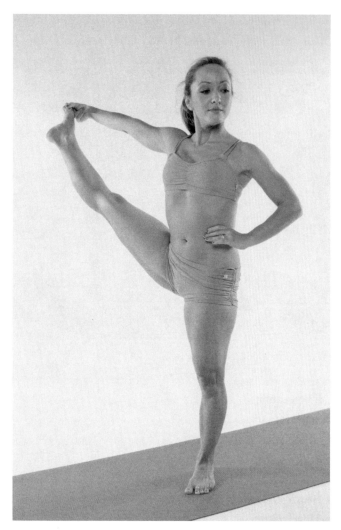

Figure 6.21

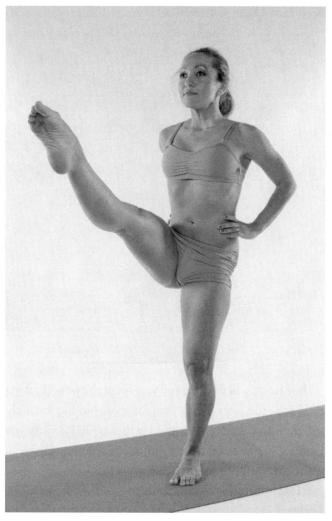

Figure 6.22

Enter Utthita Hasta Padangusthasana C directly from B. Inhale as you slowly bring your right leg back to the center, still holding your toe and controlling the movement from within your hip joint. Exhale as you fold forward once more, then inhale as you release your big toe and balance with your hands on your waist, your right leg extended in front of you (see fig. 6.22). This is the first pose that teaches you how to lift and extend while engaging and activating. Your leg must hold itself up and simultaneously remain connected with your pelvis and core muscles. The hip joint in the extended leg must remain spacious and powerful at the same time. The hamstring must extend while the quadriceps engage to help support the leg. Since the right leg lifts only to the extent that you thrust the left into the ground, attempting to lift your right leg will also help you feel the effect of gravity. Pulling the head of the femur deeper into the hip socket will also help the leg lift higher. Held for five breaths, this pose is crucial in developing the strength you need to perform the remaining portion of the Primary Series safely. When you are finished, exhale and return to Samasthiti, then repeat all three poses on the left side.

BENEFITS

Improves balance
Strengthens the legs, ankles, and core muscles
Stretches the backs of legs
Builds mental concentration

ARDHA BADDHA PADMOTTANASANA
Bound Lotus Forward Fold Pose
Drishti: Nasagrai (Nose)

Ardha Baddha Padmottanasana is primarily a balancing pose meant to teach you how to maintain stability while moving your body through space. The hardest part of this pose is finding your way safely into half-lotus position before folding forward. Many students rush into this position and end up with an injury. Since this is the first time in the practice that your body is asked to enter a lotus position, give it time and space to release and open into the pose.

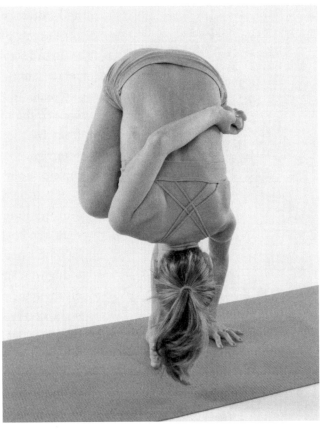

Figure 6.23

If you are a beginner or have tighter hips, start off in a modification pose where you stand with your instep pressed into the inner thigh of the standing leg in a simple Vrksasana, or Tree Pose (see fig. 6.24). Enter Tree Pose from Samasthiti (see fig. 5.1) by bending your right knee, transferring weight onto the left side, and externally rotating your right hip. Reach down with your hands and lift the right foot as close to the groin as possible. This creates a gentle, noninvasive outward movement that uses gravity's downward pull on the bent knee to deepen the lotus position. Practicing a standing half-lotus position before you try a seated half-lotus position is helpful because when you're standing, gravity opens your hip joints without muscular activation. There is also more space around your hip joints when you are standing, which gives you more freedom to move and negotiate with your pelvis. If you are using the modification, stay in it for at least five breaths to allow your hip joint to open before proceeding into the half-lotus position. You may find it useful to stand in the half-lotus for a few extra breaths before moving fully into the pose.

Regardless of your level of expertise, always enter lotus position with an outward rotation of your hip joint to prevent your knees from being injured. Use the full rotation in your hip to free up space in your pelvis

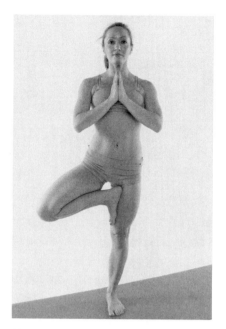

Figure 6.24

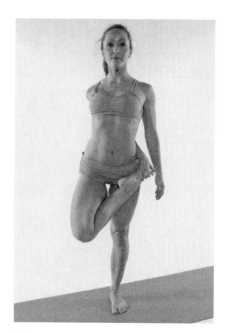

Figure 6.25

and create the room to fold forward. You should fold forward only when the knee that is in half-lotus is pointing toward the ground.

In order to get safely into half-lotus position from standing, externally rotate your right hip joint. Feel the movement in the ball and socket of the hip joint. You can do this movement while lifting your leg, bringing your knee to the side, and reaching for your foot. Or you can enter half-lotus from Tree Pose and reach down with your hands to hold on to the top of your right foot. When entering half-lotus, aim the top of your foot to the hip crease and use the full rotation in your hips.

If you are relatively flexible, you may be able to move directly into half-lotus position on the first inhalation, holding your right foot with your right hand behind your back (see fig. 6.25). Once you are in a full bound half-lotus position, exhale and fold forward while stabilizing your left leg, lifting your sit bones, and drawing in your abdomen. Place your left hand on the floor and align your fingers with your toes (see fig. 6.23). Try to maintain the structural integrity of your body by equalizing your hips and reaching your chin toward your left shin. If you lose your balance or cannot bind your lotus, you can place both hands on the floor.

Stay in the pose for five breaths. Inhale as you look up, then exhale and hold that position as you settle your weight back into your hips. Finally inhale and return to a standing position, dropping your right foot back to the floor. Repeat the pose with your left leg in half-lotus position.

BENEFITS

Teaches balance
Strengthens the legs, ankles, and core muscles
Stretches the hips and ankles
Builds mental concentration
Helps relieve symptoms of flat feet
Improves digestion
Stimulates the abdominal organs

UTKATASANA

Chair Pose

Drishti: Angustha Ma Dyai (Thumbs)

When entering the next series of three poses, you will flow through a kind of Sun Salutation to enter and exit the postures. This is the first time you will fully experience the dynamic power of the vinyasa method that co-ordinates breath with movement to enter a posture. Just as in the Surya Namaraskara, you will flow through poses linked together with the breath and hold only at specific points. Starting in Samasthiti, inhale and raise your hands as in Surya Namaskara A; exhale, fold forward. Inhale, look up and exhale, jump back to Chaturanga Dandasana. Inhale to Upward-Facing Dog, exhale to Downward-Facing Dog, and then inhale as your feet jump forward in between your hands directly into Utkatasana. Hold this for five breaths.

Stand with your feet together so the bases of your big toes and your heels touch. Your arms are raised above in line with the shoulder joints, your shoulders are drawn down your back, and your spine reaches upward. The spine is in a slightly extended position but not overarched. If you feel a strain in your lower back, you are overarched and need to straighten up a little. Bend your knees toward the front of your feet. Try to bend deeply enough that your thighs reach toward being parallel to the ground, but be conscious of the position of your spine and keep your heels on the floor. Bend only as far as you can while keeping your spine in a relatively erect and upright position. Do not overarch your back to compensate for the bend in your knees. The purpose of this asana is to build strength in your thighs, back muscles, and shoulders while keeping your body in a healthy alignment. Your wish to achieve an end result should never compromise the integrity of the pose.

Draw your stomach in to help deepen the bend inside your hip joints and give you a greater sense of ease in your body. Keep your tailbone in a neutral position or even slightly tucked to help create a sense of support from your pelvis. Raise your arms, press your elbows toward each other, and bring your shoulder blades down your back to create spaciousness around your neck and provide the structural support needed from your upper back and shoulder girdle for healthy upper body alignment (see fig. 6.26).

The tradition of gazing toward the thumbs straight up above your head is meant to give you a sense of lift throughout the pose and to direct energy up your spine. Your body should not sag downward; it should rise upward. Think of it this way: As you press down into your feet, your energy travels into the ground below. With equal and opposing force, the ground thrusts the energy back up into you, and because you are grounded, you achieve a natural lift. Once this energy begins to flow, all you have to do is let it rise naturally through your healthfully aligned body. Any kinks in your energy system will stop the flow of energy, so it is important to maintain as good an alignment as possible and to relax in the pose so the energy can flow freely. Raising your arms above your heart naturally challenges your

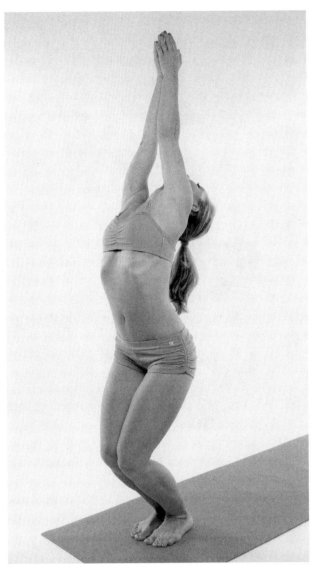

Figure 6.26

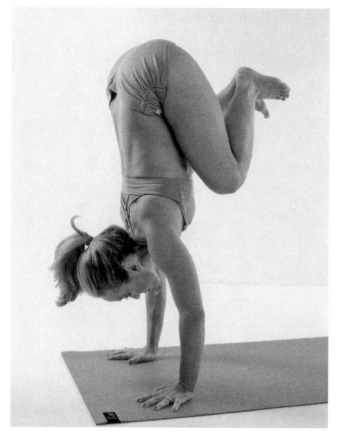

Figure 6.27

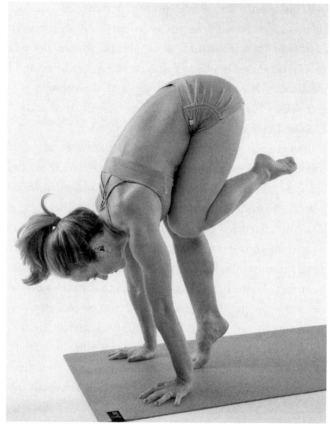

Figure 6.28

cardiovascular system and stimulates circulation throughout your body. Approach this pose with care and consideration, being careful not to over-strain your back but at the same time pushing your boundaries just enough to make steady progress.

After five breaths in this position, exhale and take your hands to the floor, while keeping the knees bent. The traditional method for exiting the pose is to place your hands firmly on the ground and lift your legs into a hovering position (see fig. 6.27). This demands great strength and took me many years to be able to integrate into my practice. An intermediary step is to bring one knee into your chest and then jump the other into your chest on an inhalation (see fig. 6.28).

Achieving balance in the hovering position is not easy and requires a great deal of practice. Your pelvis must be balanced over the solid founda-tion of your arms and your pelvic floor engaged to lift the weight of the body up. When you are attempting this movement by lifting one knee into your chest and jumping the feet into the hovering position, think about sending the weight of your body over your hands. Engage your deltoids, latissimus dorsi, serratus anterior, pelvic floor, and breathe deeply. Look down at your mat. This pose is held for only one breath so do not overexert yourself. If it doesn't happen immediately, jump back and continue the practice.

Whether you are lifting or jumping up, exhale as you jump back to Chaturanga Dandasana, inhale as you enter Urdhva Mukha Svanasana, and exhale as you go into Adho Mukha Svanasana to complete the movement.

BENEFITS

Strengthens the knees, calves, ankles, and spine
Stretches the Achilles tendon
Stimulates digestion, circulation, and the cardio-
vascular system
Lifts the arches of the feet
Aligns the pelvis and spine
Deepens awareness of the hip joint

VIRABHADRASANA A AND B

Warrior I and II

Drishti: Hastagrai (Fingers)

Continue in flow immediately after one breath in Adho Mukha Svanasana and begin to enter this pose, starting on the right side just as in Surya Namaskara B. Begin by holding Downward-Facing Dog while rotating your left hip joint externally and turning your left foot out between forty-five and ninety degrees (depending on your hip flexibility). Step your right foot forward between your hands and align the right heel with the left arch if possible (or align the heels with each other if you are a beginner). When your legs are in position, lift your torso so that it is stacked directly on top of the pelvic bowl, raise your arms over your head, drop your shoulder blades down your back, and gaze at your fingers. This entire movement should be done on one long inhalation, but if you need extra breaths to coordinate, remember to always coordinate your breath with your movement.

Virabhadrasana A is a great pose to help build your alignment and strength for backbends later and for preparing your hip joints for the outward rotation that makes lotus position easy (see fig. 6.29). Turn your left foot outward as close to ninety degrees as possible and align your left heel with your right arch. Bend your right knee until it is at least over your ankle but ideally over the middle of your foot. If you have a hard time knowing how much to bend your knee, focus on feeling your legs underneath

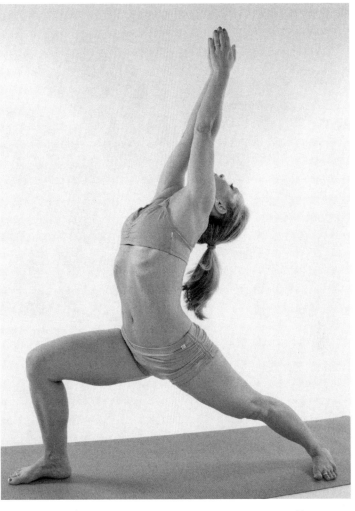

Figure 6.29

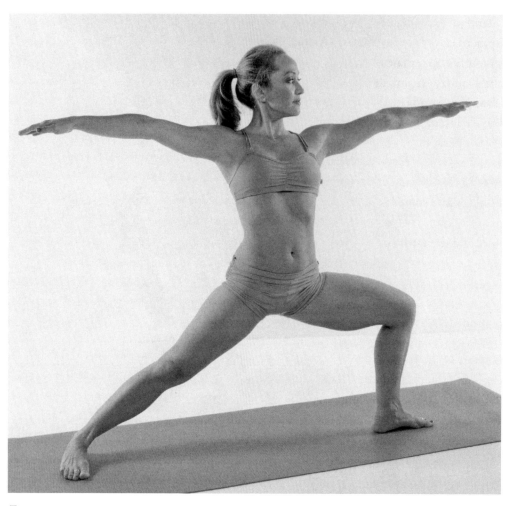

Figure 6.30

you and strengthening your quadriceps, but do not let your knee extend past your toes. Your feet should be spread far enough apart so that when you bend your knee over your foot, your thigh is parallel to the ground. Finding the perfect distance is unique to each person's height and body proportions, so be careful of simply mirroring your teacher or another practitioner. Always check in with your own body.

As you bend your right knee, keep your left leg straight and your hip joint level as your right leg rotates slightly inward and left leg rotates outward. Keep your pelvis pointing forward toward your right knee as much as possible to ensure that your left hip joint is actually rotating outward. Be careful not to twist your left knee and force your left foot to turn out too far. Pay attention to the range of motion in your hip joint. Make sure the outer edge of your back foot is firmly planted into the ground and the arches of both feet are lifted. Squaring your hips to the center as much as possible once your forward knee is deeply bent will stretch your psoas muscles (on the sides of your lower back) and hip flexors, opening up the front of your pelvis. This opening is crucial for backbends.

Keep your tailbone in a neutral position, and ignore the temptation to stick it out and overarch your lower back. This is an excellent opportunity to retrain your body to keep your tailbone in a neutral position while opening your hip flexors, psoas muscles, and hip joints. Over time, the "flipped-out" tailbone position compresses your lower back, sacroiliac joints, and the whole back of your pelvis, and is not a sustainable method of movement for long-term practice because it lacks support for your spine. Whenever you have a pattern of movement that leads to pain, it is best to retrain your body to use a better pattern whenever the old pattern arises.

Once you have the solid foundation of your legs, draw your abdomen in and lift the floor of your pelvis in and up. Activate your back muscles (erector spinae) to help lift each vertebra up and away from your pelvis. Do not hang down in the natural extension and flexibility of the lumbar spine. Instead, build your extension and strength to create space between each joint by actively lifting your spine up and away from your pelvis while drawing your stomach in to support the movement from the front. This muscular pattern actually helps bring energy up your spine and the central column of your body, thereby increasing the spiritual energy of the pose. You practice this action here so that you have the strength for deeper backbends later.

When the energy reaches your chest, draw your shoulder blades down your back and away from each other, lifting your arms over your head, opening your shoulder girdle, and creating space around your neck. Keep your spine in a natural position and do not overarch your upper back. Lift your sternum up and slightly forward while straightening your arms. Press your hands flat against each other, engage your deltoids, and press your elbows toward each other. Bringing your arms over your head encourages your heart to pump more vigorously, thereby increasing the strength of your cardiovascular system. Tilt your head back and gaze steadily at your thumbs; try not to interlock your fingers. Rotate your shoulders externally to build the strength and flexibility needed to stabilize your body in more challenging asanas such as handstands and backbends. Hold the pose for five breaths, then inhale as you pivot your feet and exhale to enter the pose on the left. Hold the left side for five breaths. Do not come up to standing in between. Keep your arms raised as you switch sides.

Virabhadrasana B uses the same foot alignment as A (see fig. 6.30). Move into this variation by turning your hips away from your bent knee, opening your arms out to the sides, and inhaling. You will start off on the left side. Be careful to keep your left knee in the same position over your ankle. Actively draw your tailbone in to counteract any feelings of overarching so you end up in a neutral position. Send your pelvis away from your left knee so your pubic bone is at a ninety-degree angle from that knee. Rotate both legs outward and dig lower down into your legs and hip joints.

This version of the pose is meant to open your groin and inner thigh muscles while continuing to build muscular strength to lift your spine. Your tailbone remains grounded while your spine lifts away from the foundation underneath. Roll your shoulder blades down your back and away from each other, keeping your arms extended to the sides at shoulder height. Gaze at the fingers of your left hand. There is a tendency here to let the back arm sag, so remember to reach toward the front and back equally. Keep your torso stacked over your pelvis so your spine is in a neutral but lifted position. Do not lean forward or sideways with your torso; instead, find balance and peace in the pose.

Hold the pose for five breaths, then exhale and pivot to the right to repeat the pose. After five breaths on the right side, exhale and take your hands to ground. Place your right hand on the floor on the outside of your right foot and your left hand on the floor on the inside of your right foot. Keep the right knee bent as you spin forward onto the ball of the left foot, bringing the hips into parallel position. If you have good upper body strength, float forward onto your arms and come to a balance point. Your legs will remain in the same position as you shift your straight left leg and your bent right knee over your arms. Then exhale and jump back to Chaturanga Dandasana. Beginners should skip that movement and simply step back to Chaturanga Dandasana from the moment that both hands are on the floor and the hips are in parallel position.

Remember to exhale as you enter Chaturanga Dandasana, inhale as you go into Urdhva Mukha Svanasana, and exhale as you enter Adho Mukha Svanasana to complete the movement.

BENEFITS

Strengthens the leg muscles, especially the quadriceps
Stretches the psoas muscles, hip flexors, and groin
Prepares the body for backbends
Opens the shoulders and heart
Cleanses the cardiovascular system

7

Seated Poses: Grow Your Lotus

THE ASANAS THAT ARE EXCLUSIVE TO THE ASHTANGA Yoga Primary Series are mostly seated poses. The logic is that the Surya Namaskaras and standing poses build a sense of connection with the earth, the dynamics of movement, and the inner body. Once this is established, you enter a wide variety of twists, forward bends, hip rotations, strength poses, and backbends. The practical experience of the core strength work you need to sustain healthy alignment throughout these later poses is more readily available when you can thrust into the floor. In the seated poses, you must thrust into the soles of your feet and replicate the same energetic connection as you would if your feet were fully planted on the floor. With a firm sense of balance, spatial orientation, inner stability, and flexibility, you can move into the seated poses with confidence and ease.

These poses are grouped into related series. They also build to a midpoint crescendo of challenging external rotation that involves placing both legs behind your head. Just the sound of that may send you running; it's one of the yoga exercises that the average person thinks only a contortionist can do. But the Ashtanga Yoga Primary Series trains your body slowly, preparing it step-by-step for deep and complex movements. When you perform the seated poses with sound anatomical knowledge as a guide, you will experience the increased openness you need to enter all poses safely.

The second group of seated poses helps release your spine, strengthen your erector spinae muscles, and build a steady transition into backbends. Taken together, the seated poses work your entire body. You will open your hip joints to prepare for full lotus position and legs behind your head, build the core strength needed for arm balances, and work your spine and shoulders in preparation for backbends.

The emotional lesson of the seated poses is a kind of turning inward of the body and mind. It is a deeply balancing and healing practice that cleanses the digestive system of old toxins and encourages a conscious state of self-reflection. This practice allows the mind to maintain unbroken focus on the inner body rather than being directed outward. The seated poses seek to concentrate your energy and refine your body. If you approach these poses with respect and patience, you can master them. Since many of the seated poses target either the right or left side, you will notice that one hip joint, shoulder, or side of your body is tighter. This is totally normal, and there is no reason to fear the pose or your body. You may find it useful to stay in position longer on the tighter side while breathing deeply, but do not expect symmetry from your body. Practice with patience and acceptance, knowing that the full benefits of the practice are spiritual and cannot be measured by your physical performance.

DANDASANA

Staff Pose

Drishti: Nasagrai (Nose)

Dandasana plays a crucial role in the development of healthy forward bends and sets up your technique and knowledge of anatomy for deeper movements that support your lower back, build core strength, and elongate your hamstrings. This pose is not traditionally identified while practicing Ashtanga Yoga, and many students overlook it; however, it is like the seated version of Samsthiti, a neutral position used to enter all other poses.

Inhale as you jump through your arms from Adho Mukha Svanasana to a seated position. Students unfamiliar with the transitions between seated poses known as "jumping through" and "jumping back" (the vinyasa) should reference Chapter 10. Exhale as you sit up as straight as possible, place your hands flat on the floor next to your hips, and straighten your legs. If you have long arms, you will need to bend them slightly to keep your shoulder girdle relaxed. If your arms are short, your hands may not touch floor, so be careful not to round your back and force your hands to the floor. Keep your shoulder girdle broad and open, drop your shoulder blades down your back, and lift your chest. Tuck your chin under; as you inhale, your sternum will rise toward your chin and ideally touch. As you exhale, your chest drops, and your chin and chest separate (see fig. 7.1).

Be sure that you bend at the waist from the hip joints and keep your spine erect while extending your legs out at a ninety-degree angle. Engage your legs by thrusting your heels away from your pelvis and into the "ground" while lifting your kneecaps and activating your inner quadriceps. Imagine a floor under your feet and connect to it through your legs from the bases of your big toes along your quadriceps and all the way into your pelvic floor. To build core strength and protect the hamstring attachments, thrust your sit bones into the floor and actively push downward to engage your pelvic floor. Consciously work these muscles and suck in your abdomen to create more access to the interior space of your pelvis. Draw your belly (from your navel down to your pubic bone) in as much as possible to support a natural lift of your spine. Be careful not to overarch or round your lumbar spine. Instead, allow the core muscles to support a natural lumbar curve. Bring your attention to your erector

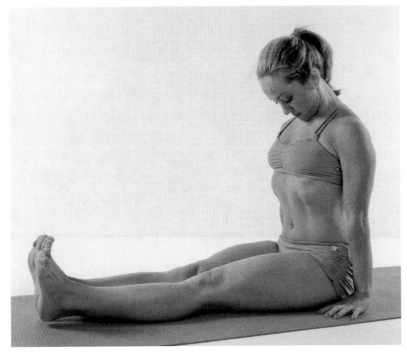

Figure 7.1

spinae muscles, think about sending your spine upward, and lift it out of your pelvis to create space between each vertebra. Let your energy reach out through the top of your head but remain grounded to the floor with the support of your sit bones. Your breath should travel up and down the inner regions of your spine but not go into your lower stomach. At no time during this pose should you push your belly out. In fact, drawing it in is the key to setting up the most healthy use of your spine in all later forward bends.

If you are unable to sit with an erect spine and have a severely rounded lower back, you may find it useful to bend your knees slightly so you can gain access to your hip joints. If you must bend your knees, make a conscious effort to straighten them as much as possible while maintaining both the lift in your spine and the natural curvature of your lumbar region. If you are more advanced, you may be able to send your heels away from your pelvis and lift them slightly off the ground. As long as the backs of your knees are not thrusting into the ground and your knees are not hyperextended, this movement is useful. Hold the pose for five breaths, then move immediately into the next pose, Paschimattanasana.

BENEFITS

Aligns the pelvis and hips
Strengthens awareness of the central axis
Builds the bandhas
Strengthens the legs

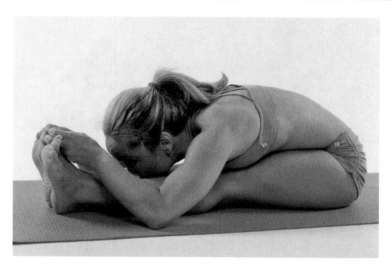

Figure 7.2

PASCHIMATTANASANA A AND D

Seated Forward Bend A and D

Drishti: Padhayoragrai (Toes)

Begin in Dandasana. Apply the three components of forward bends — lengthening the backs of your legs from the sit bones to the heels, drawing in your abdomen, and elongating your back muscles — presented in the standing poses. Although there is a slightly different activation pattern here, the same alignment rules apply. Instead of thrusting into the ground, you must re-create the sensation of the floor under your feet by pushing the bases of your big toes together (which causes your thighs to rotate in slightly) and actively engaging the soles of your feet. Press your heels into the floor if you feel pain at the hamstring attachment or reach them slightly away from your pelvis if you can go deeper. All forward bends involve a slight flexing of the spine, so it is crucial to have the support of your core muscles by drawing in your abdomen to protect your spine from injury and maximize the spaciousness between your joints.

Instead of surrendering your back to gravity to elongate it, as in standing poses, use the inner muscles of your torso to create the same spaciousness and length. Inhale as you consciously suck in your lower belly (drawing the area between your pubic bone and navel deeply into your body), lengthen your spine, and fold forward to grab your big toes. Exhale to deepen the bend into full Paschimattanasana A (see fig. 7.2). Be careful not to tense your abdominal muscles, or you will merely create muscular tension that will prevent you from going deeply into the pose. The healing and cleansing aspect of this deep forward fold comes from pulling in your abdomen and cleaning out your digestive system.

The same activation of the legs as in Dandasana applies here, so reach from deep inside your pelvis to feel a long line of energy traveling from your hip joints through your lifted kneecaps and activated inner quadriceps to a firm floor under your flexed feet. If you had to bend your knees to modify Dandasana, you will need the same modification here, but try to straighten your legs as much as possible by thrusting your feet away from your pelvis. If you have a hamstring injury, you can either press your sit bones and heels into the ground or, if that does not relieve the pain, bend your knees slightly until the injury heals.

Be careful not to pull too hard with your upper body. Allow the work of the forward bend to happen deep within your pelvis and body. Use your inner body to lengthen from within. Keep your shoulders open and only slightly active. Breathe into your lungs and allow the energy to flow freely throughout your entire body. Hold the pose for five breaths.

Inhale and lift your spine, then exhale as you take the deepest grip possible around your feet; hold your toes again, interlace your fingers around your feet, hold the outsides of your feet, or grab your wrist. Inhale again to create space, then exhale as you hold Paschimattanasana D for another five breaths (see fig. 7.3).

There are four different version of Paschimattanasana, but the present Ashtanga Yoga method uses only two: the introductory one and the last, deepest version. If you have more time to practice or you find forward bends difficult, you may want to proceed through all four variations. Consult *Yoga Mala* for further details.

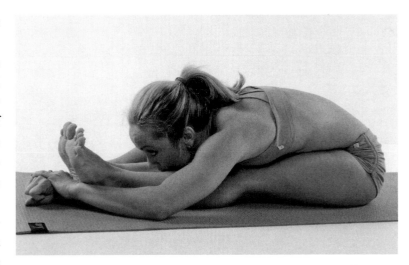

Figure 7.3

After five breaths in Paschimattanasana D, inhale and lift your spine while maintaining your grip; exhale as you settle your weight into your hips and lift your pelvic floor even deeper. Inhale, release your grip, and lift up; exhale and jump back. (The Ashtanga Yoga jump back and jump through movements are explained in greater detail in Chapter 10.)

BENEFITS

Improves digestion
Stretches the hamstrings
Treats sciatica
Cleanses the internal organs

PURVATTANASANA

Upward-Facing Plank Pose

Drishti: Broomadhya (Eyebrow center)

When practiced with Dandasana and Paschimattanasana, this pose completes the full range of movement in the spine by extending it. This technique prepares the body for backbends and helps relieve any pressure on the spine after the deep forward fold in Paschimattanasana. Inhale as you jump through to a seated position, and exhale as you set up the pose. Roll your spine under until your sacrum is on the ground, suck in your abdomen, and move your hands behind you so your hands are about a foot away from your pelvis and flat on the floor. Point your fingers toward your feet and inhale as you lift up (see fig. 7.5).

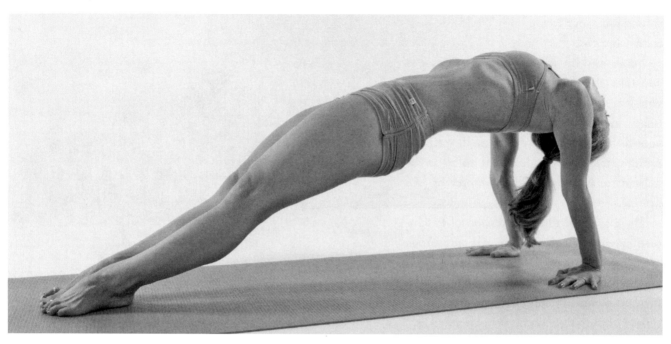

Figure 7.4

Rotate your thighs and hip joints inward to create a long line of energy throughout both legs. Just as in the previous two poses, engage your inner quadriceps firmly and connect your actively lifted kneecaps both to your pelvic floor and to your toes. Point your toes firmly and press the bases of your big toes together to complete the energetic reach of the inward rotation.

Press your toes into the floor to help engage your legs and lift your pelvis. The inward rotation of the hip joints and thighs relieves pressure on the lower back and sacrum.

Send your pelvis and tailbone strongly forward and nutate your sacrum to arch your lower back slightly and lift up. This pose should be a backbend, so use the natural extension of your spine to go deeper. Allow your erector spinae muscles to support your body from underneath. Be especially careful not to push out your abdomen while lifting. Instead, keep it drawn in, sucking your stomach muscles in toward your spine. If your stomach pooches out, then the weight of your organs will fall down into the open vertebrae, endangering the discs, so keep your lower belly drawn in.

Once you have established the foundation of the pose with strong legs and active lifting of the pelvis, you can concentrate on your upper body. Lift your chest high, and open the center of your heart toward the ceiling. Engage your arms strongly by pressing into the floor through your fingertips; straighten your arms. Drop your head backward, but be careful to support your neck. Draw your shoulder blades down your back to support the lift through your upper back (see fig. 7.4). As this is a backbend, you use every muscle in your body; every vertebra along your spinal column must extend, create space, and ultimately use that space to bend. Breathe consciously and deeply. After five breaths, exhale and come down. Inhale and lift up; exhale and jump back.

BENEFITS

Strengthens and extends the back
Counters forward bends
Treats fatigue

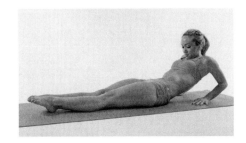

Figure 7.5

ARDHA BADDHA PADMA PASCHIMATTANASANA

Half-Bound Lotus Forward Bend

Drishti: Padhayoragrai (Toes)

This is the first seated pose that challenges your external rotation and tests the awareness and openness of the hip joint movement you learned in the standing poses. It demands full attention, care, and patience. This is an excellent place to work on understanding and integrating the principles of healthy external rotation and developing your lotus position. Some people need to stop here before proceeding if their hip joints are too tight; otherwise, the chance of injury may be increased in later poses.

Inhale as you jump through to a seated position from Downward-Facing Dog in the vinyasa after Purvattanasana. If you are an advanced practitioner, exhale as you take your right foot into half-lotus position. Hold your foot with your right hand around your back. Hold the outside of your left foot with your left hand and align your sternum forward over your left knee. Do all of this on the same inhalation as you used to get through, set up, and prepare. Then exhale and fold forward to fully enter the pose (see fig. 7.6).

If you are a beginner, you will do well to slow that movement and break it down into manageable bits. Start by rotating your right hip joint and pointing your knee out to the side. Bend your right knee to close the joint and bring the sole of your right foot to your left inner thigh. Lift your right foot and right knee gently off the ground and use the external rotation of the hip joint to aim your right foot toward your left hip crease. If you feel pain in your right knee, back off and dial down the level of rotation in your hip joint. As you are getting into the pose, avoid twisting your knee joint; if possible, use the external spiraling motion of your hip joint to get into the pose. If your knee is floating off the floor, do not push it down and do not tense the muscles around it. If you are able to rotate your hip joint and place your foot in the appropriate position but you feel pain in your knee, you may find it useful to rest your right knee on a block or a towel to give it appropriate support.

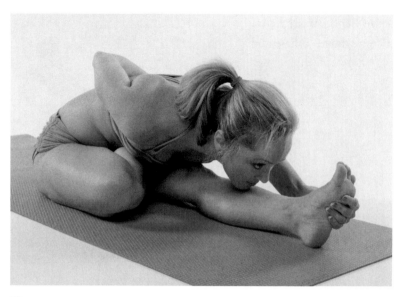

Figure 7.6

As a general note for how to practice, if you feel pain in one area of your body, the immediate response is often fear. Try to put yourself in a state of mind to experience the pain instead of just running from it. For example, if you feel pain, be as specific as possible about its epicenter, the type of pain, and what your emotional response is. We often feel pain in a general area, but the more specific we can be about where and what it actually is, the less we fear it and the more we can work with it in our practice and our lives. If you feel pain in the joint, back off immediately, but if the muscles are burning and stretching, you can proceed with caution and attention to alignment.

If all goes well with the half-lotus position, reach your right hand around your back using the full rotation of your shoulder to hold the top of your right foot. Try not to twist your body too much in order to grasp your foot; instead, let the movement come from your shoulder and upper back as your shoulder blade descends along your back. Once you clasp your right foot, firmly engage your shoulder and pull your torso back to center to counterbalance any twisting it may have done to allow you to reach your foot. If possible, engage your right foot and press the heel into the interior space of your pelvis. This will encourage you to draw your abdomen in and increase the suction of the bandhas, as explained in Chapter 10.

Inhale as you reach forward and hold on to the outside edge of your left foot. If possible, draw your left shoulder blade down your back and square your chest so that your sternum and pubic bone follow the same, central line as the rest of your body. As you exhale, reach your chin to your left shin and hold for five breaths.

This is a complicated motion that often requires additional breaths to allow the body to open. Be patient, and do not rush the movement at all. If you need to stop at any point during the movement and hold your maximum limit of flexibility, absolutely follow the advice of your body. Never squeeze your knee; always allow its movement to originate in the hip joint.

After five breaths, inhale and lift your spine while still maintaining your hold on both feet. Exhale, keep hold of your feet, settle into the pose, and catch hold of the strength of the pelvis to prepare for the vinyasa. Inhale and lift up; exhale and jump back; complete the vinyasa; inhale and jump through; then repeat the pose on the opposite side.

BENEFITS

Increases digestion and awareness of the
bandhas
Stretches the hamstrings, hips, and shoulders
Cleanses the internal organs

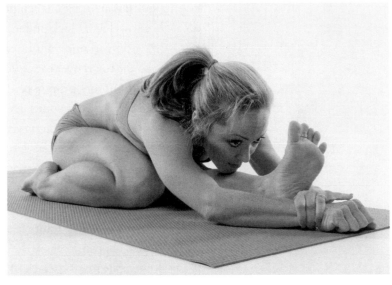

TIRYANG MUKHA EKAPADA PASCHIMATTANASANA

Three-Limbed Forward Fold Pose

Drishti: Padhayoragrai (Toes)

While the majority of poses in the Primary
Series use an external rotation of the hip joint,

Figure 7.7

this one uses an internal rotation of that joint. Most people think the top
of the thigh needs to rise in order to turn the thigh inward, but the head of
the thighbone actually still reaches back and down while it rotates deeply
inside the ball and socket of the hip joint. The key to easy internal rotation
is to widen the sacrum, freeing space along the back of the body and allowing the thighs to come closer together.

Inhale as you jump through to a seated position from Downward Dog
after the last vinyasa for Ardha Baddha Padma Paschimattanasana. Bend
your right knee backward, rotate your thighs inward, and point your right
foot away from the left. Leave enough space between your right foot and
your pelvis so that your right hip can sink to the floor. You may find it helpful to move your right calf muscle out of the way to create more space for
your knee to bend. To prepare, inhale as you grip your wrist as far as possible around your left foot or simply hold the foot with both hands if you
are unable to hold on to the wrist. Exhale as you begin folding forward
along the centerline of your body, keeping your knees as close together
as possible. Reach your chin toward your left shin, but do not shift your
weight forward or to the left (see fig. 7.7).

Draw your lower belly in and engage your pelvic floor to create the stable
support you need to move deeply into the pose. Engage your left foot and
send energy into the floor through the heel and out through the base of
the big toe. Press your left calf muscle into the ground to push energy back
into your pelvis and help ground your right sit bone. While most people
feel the right sit bone rise off the ground, try your best to send energy
down through the interior space of your pelvis to keep it rooted toward the
ground. Feel the head of your femur on the right side moving deeper into the
hip socket.

If you find it challenging to keep your knee bent, you may want to place a towel or a block under the opposite hip to elevate your pelvis and release tension around your knee. If you begin by using the block, try to graduate to the towel over the course of a year or two, then finally try doing the pose without any prop over the course of another year or two. If you feel an intense pain in your knees when in this pose, it may stem from either lack of internal rotation or very tight quadriceps. If you feel a sharp pain at the center of the knee, back off and modify the pose with a block. Proceed with caution and do not force your body into any pose. Instead, allow the pose to unfold over time with patience and deep breathing.

Bringing your torso over your thighs while encouraging an inward rotation of the hip joints is a crucial preparation for the deep twisting poses that happen later in the series. If you have a hard time twisting, part of the issue may be a lack of internal hip rotation, and this is the perfect pose to help remedy that. Hold the pose for five breaths, then inhale and lift your spine, exhale and settle into the pose. Inhale, place your hands on the ground, and lift up. Exhale to jump back, and complete the vinyasa. Inhale to jump through, and repeat the pose on the opposite side.

BENEFITS

Increases digestion and awareness of the bandhas
Internally rotates the hip joints
Cleanses the internal organs
Deepens awareness of the inner body

JANU SIRSASANA A

Head-to-Knee Pose A

Drishti: Padhayoragrai (Toes)

Janu Sirsasana A allows you to open your hips, inner thighs, and back safely and easily while strengthening your core. Inhale and jump through to a seated position from Downward-Facing Dog following the last vinyasa of Tiryang Mukha Ekapada Paschimattanasana. Externally rotate your right hip joint, pointing your knee out to the side at ninety degrees. Relax the hip joint as you allow the ball and socket to open and release. As the joint opens and allows you to move deeper into it, you will be able to bend your right knee freely and close the knee joint fully. Do not rush the movement; listen to your body every step of the way.

The deepest version of this pose has the outer edge of the sole of your right foot resting against your inner left thigh and your right heel resting close to your pubic bone. To keep the movement out of your knee and in your hip, be sure to rotate the head of your thighbone back and down, rolling your upper thigh toward the back of your pelvis while elongating your inner thigh muscles. Once this external rotation is established, turn your pelvis as far forward as possible and align your torso over your left thigh so your heart and sternum are centered forward toward your left knee and in alignment with your pubic bone. Grip your wrist around your left foot (or hold your left foot with both hands) and straighten your arms as you inhale. Exhale to fold forward and reach your chin to your left shin.

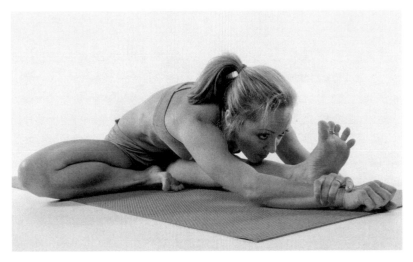

Figure 7.8

Keep your torso lifting up and away from your pelvis by drawing in your abdomen, engaging your pelvic floor, and stretching your back muscles. Direct your gaze gently toward the toes on your left foot (see fig. 7.8). Since you are working your body in at least two directions — back and down with the hip and forward and away with your torso — this pose increases coordination and brain function. The action of drawing in your lower belly also helps purify the interior space of your pelvis and your digestive system. Opening the inner thigh helps cleanse the kidney meridians.

If you are a beginner or have tighter hip joints, you may find it useful to close the knee only partially and allow it to hover slightly off the ground with a block or towel placed under it for support. As your hip joint opens, remove the prop. If you feel pain inside the knee joint, back off a little by leaving the sole of your right foot closer to your left knee than to the upper inner thigh. If you can bend your knee fully but it is still off the floor, you are safe as long as there is no pain.

One other modification to help alleviate pain in the knee is to roll your right thigh inward toward the front of your pelvis instead of outward. This lessens the rotation and can sometimes relieve pressure in the knee. Try both options if you find the pose difficult and build up to the full pose over many years of practice. After five long, deep breaths on the right side, inhale and straighten your spine, then exhale and settle into the movement. Inhale and lift up; exhale and jump back. Repeat the pose on the opposite side.

If you are a total beginner and have advanced this far in the seated poses, you might want to stop here and get used to maintaining a daily practice before learning the remainder of the seated poses. You could skip the remaining seated poses and move immediately to backbends if you feel your stamina and endurance are challenged. It is better to have a shorter practice you can do more frequently than a longer practice you do only occasionally. Continuity is one of the main determinations of success in yoga practice.

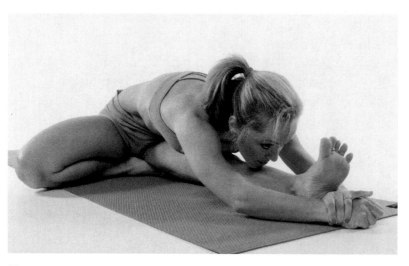

Figure 7.9

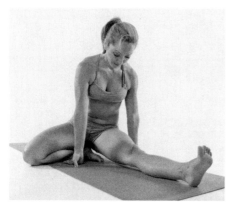

Figure 7.10

BENEFITS

Cleanses the liver, kidneys, and abdominal
    organs
Stimulates the kidney meridian
Improves digestion

JANU SIRSASANA B

Head-to-Knee Pose B

Drishti: Padhayoragrai (Toes)

Enter this pose in the same way you entered
Janu Sirsasana A, following the same vin-
yasa. Start with your right knee pointed outward at a ninety-degree angle.
Place your hands on the floor and lift your pelvis off the ground (see fig.
7.10). Push your body forward over your right foot until your pelvis rests
on top of it and your right knee points out to the side between eighty and
eighty-five degrees. Allow your perineum to make contact with the heel
of your right foot and let your weight rest there. Be sure to use the same
principles of outward rotation as in the previous pose to protect your knee
and safely enter the pose. Try to keep your right foot flexed so the toes are
pointing forward toward your left foot.

If you are a beginner, pointing your toes and bringing your knee closer
to forty-five degrees will lessen some of your discomfort. However, this
pose will always be slightly uncomfortable. After getting your right foot
into the appropriate position, align your torso forward over your left leg,
and grip your wrist around your left foot or hold on to your foot with both
hands as you inhale. Then exhale to enter the pose, folding forward toward
your left shin (see fig. 7.9).

Pressing your heel into your perineum is meant to stimulate the engagement of your pelvic floor. Awakening the energy centers in the pelvic region
and stimulating the vagus nerve induces a state of relaxation. Once you
have established the proper anatomical and technical details for your lower
body, begin aligning your torso and pubic bone along the centerline of
your body, facing forward as much as possible. Janu Sirsasana B involves
a deeper stretch through the sacrum and lower back, and it helps open
this area for deeper external rotations. Remember to support your body
by drawing in your abdomen, engaging your pelvic floor, and lifting your
torso up and away from the external rotation that grounds your pelvis.
Gaze at the toes on your left foot. If your chin cannot make contact with
your shin, you can either place your forehead on your shin and gaze at your
nose, or reach your torso forward and keep your gaze on your toes. After

five breaths, inhale and lift your spine. Exhale and settle into the pose. Inhale and lift up; exhale and jump back. Repeat the pose on the opposite side.

BENEFITS

Cleanses the liver, kidneys, and abdominal organs
Stimulates the kidney meridian
Improves digestion
Opens the sacrum

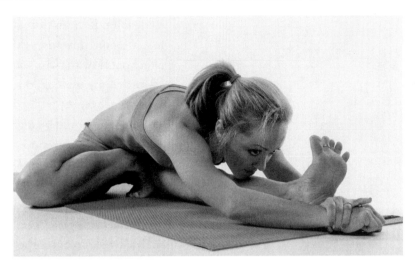

Figure 7.11

JANU SIRSASANA C

Head-to-Knee Pose C

Drishti: Padhayoragrai (Toes)

This is one of the poses in the Ashtanga Yoga sequence that seems a little scary when you first approach it. While you do want to proceed with caution, this is a safe and effective pose if practiced with awareness.

Inhale, and jump through to a seated position from Downward-Facing Dog after the last vinyasa in Janu Sirsasana B. Begin by moving into Janu Sirsasana A, closing your right knee joint totally and externally rotating your hip joint to the fullest extent. Soften your knee and place no tension around the muscles that support it. Lift your whole right leg off the ground while keeping the knee bent and closed. Flex your right foot strongly but keep your knee soft; increase the external rotation and movement in your right hip joint. Grip the base of your toes by interlacing your right hand around your ankle so you are holding your foot underneath your ankle. Twist your foot by opening the Achilles tendon and ankle joint, and place all five toes on the ground as close to your left thigh as possible. Point your heel up, slightly back, and to the left. Support the instep of your right foot on your inner left thigh. Keep your toes and ankle engaged, and support the pose with the external rotation of your right hip joint and the engagement of your pelvic floor.

Once you have fully rotated your hip joint and your ankle, your right knee should be out to the side between seventy-five and eighty degrees. Do not put pressure on your knee. If you are able to keep all five toes on the floor, let go of your foot and see if your knee floats down to the ground. If it doesn't reach, do not try to force it. You may need to place a block, towel, or some other support under it. If all five toes are not on the ground, see if you can scoot your hips and pelvis forward to increase the fold in your ankle joint. If this is not possible, you may want to sit on a block when you first attempt this pose; this gives you space to rotate your hip joint and figure out how to twist your ankle without injuring your knee. Should you choose to use a block, do so for a few months and gradually lessen your dependence on it.

This pose should be slightly uncomfortable for your toes. Relax as much as possible and surrender to the experience. By entering this movement, you are stretching your ankles deeply and relieving pressure in your feet and toes. Be sure to engage your pelvic floor for support.

After twisting your ankle as much as possible, align your body forward over your left leg and grip your left foot or clasp your wrist around your ankle. Exhale to enter the pose, folding forward over your left thigh (see fig. 7.11). As you bend, your right knee will move closer to the ground, but do not force your body into the movement. After five breaths, inhale and lift your spine, then exhale and settle into the pose. Inhale and lift up; exhale and jump back. Repeat the pose on the opposite side.

BENEFITS

Cleanses the liver, kidneys, and abdominal organs
Stimulates the kidney meridian
Improves digestion
Stretches the toes, Achilles tendons, and ankles

MARICHASANA A

Pose Dedicated to Sage Marichi A

Drishti: Padhayoragrai (Toes)

This is the first in a series of four poses named after the Indian sage Marichi, son of Brahma, who could create life with the power of his mind. It is said that by practicing poses named after a sage, you get the qualities of that particular person. Marichi is also considered to be the progenitor of the Vedic Adam, or father of humanity, so it is no wonder that so many poses are named after him. There are, in fact, four additional poses named after Marichi in the Ashtanga Yoga Fourth Series. All of them involve either forward bends or twists from a seated position while you attempt to keep your pelvis as stable and level as possible.

To enter Marichasana A, inhale as you jump through to a seated position from Downward-Facing Dog after the last vinyasa in Janu Sirsasana C. Bend your right knee and place the sole of your right foot flat on the floor about a hand's distance away from your left thigh. Bend your right knee completely so the heel of your right foot is as close as possible to your right thigh, aligning your foot with the outer edge of your sit bone or the outer edge of your right hip joint. Keep your pelvis as level as possible. Bend slightly forward from the waist toward your left thigh while firmly drawing in your abdomen and pelvic floor. Reach your right arm and shoulder down around your right shin, rotating your shoulder forward, bending your elbow, and reaching your hand along the back of your body, making contact with either your right thigh or your right lower

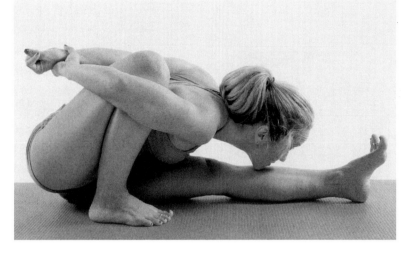

Figure 7.12

back. Reach your left arm behind your back and search for your right hand. Catch your left wrist with the right hand or interlace the fingers of both hands. If you cannot reach your fingers, hold a towel behind your back or let your fingers hover in the air. Look for the sensation of binding your fingers to close the energetic loop between your right and left hands.

Engage your shoulders by drawing your shoulder blades down your back and away from each other and stabilizing your deltoids. Square your chest and keep your shoulder girdle open. Exhale as you bend forward and place your chin on your left shin (see fig. 7.12).

Resist the temptation to let your right sit bone come off the ground too much when you bend forward. While it is okay to allow the sit bone to rise slightly, do not dump your weight forward or to the left. Instead, keep your sit bone grounded, even if you allow it to rise off the ground a little bit.

There are two crucial directions at work in the body in this pose. Your right hip joint is in a parallel position but drawn back intensely and toward the ground. You should feel your right thigh separating and pulling back from the forward direction of your torso. This movement opens your sacrum, widening it to prepare for deep hip-opening poses later, and also releases all the muscles along your lower back. The second direction is the reach of your torso forward and away toward your left thigh. This can only be achieved with a careful application of all the technical points related to forward bends that most of the preceding poses have prepared you for. Try not to round your back or worry about touching your head to your shin if you feel very tight. Instead, focus on separating your torso from your right thigh and elongating your spine forward while reaching your hips back and down. This will create the type of higher body consciousness needed to go deeper safely. Remember to coordinate each movement with a breath so that if you need more than the traditional single breath to enter and exit the pose, you always unite one breath with one movement.

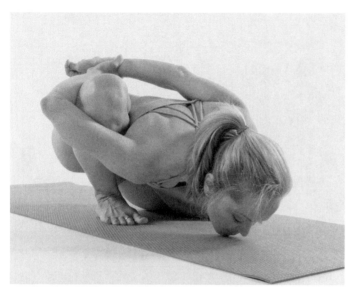

Figure 7.13

Gaze forward toward your left toes. After five breaths, inhale and straighten your spine. Exhale to settle into the pose. Inhale and lift up; exhale and jump back. Repeat the pose on the opposite side.

BENEFITS

Cleanses the liver, kidneys, and abdominal organs
Improves digestion
Opens the hips and shoulders

MARICHASANA B

Pose Dedicated to Sage Marichi B

Drishti: Nasagrai (Nose)

Marichasana B increases the challenge of opening your hip joints, sacrum, and shoulders, and it demands greater support from your lower belly and pelvic floor to enter the pose safely.

Inhale and jump through to seated position from Downward-Facing Dog after the last vinyasa in Marichasana A. Take your left leg into half-lotus position, following the movement pattern outlined in Ardha Baddha Padma Paschimattanasana. Make sure the top of your left foot is resting firmly in your hip crease, your heel is pressing into the right side of your lower abdomen, and your left knee is resting on the floor. Bend your right knee in the same fashion as in Marichasana A. As you do this, your left knee will rise off the floor slightly. Be careful not to tense your left knee; just let it be there in a relaxed and open way. If you are already challenged and find this movement hard, stay here for at least five breaths and then modify by placing your left foot underneath your right hip joint to proceed to the next step of the pose (see fig. 7.14).

With the half-lotus or a sufficient modification in place, lean your weight forward so your left knee rests firmly on the floor and your sit bones start to lift off the ground a bit. Do not dump your weight forward or to the left. Carefully shift your weight into your right big toe and heel. Just as in Marichasana A, you must work with at least two different directions: forward with your torso, and back and down with your hips. Do not be too rigid in your application of the technique; remember to explore with your body and the movement.

Once you have bent forward from the waist, reach your right arm and shoulder down around your right shin, rotating your right shoulder forward so that your hand rests gently along the back of your body, making contacting with either your right thigh or your right lower back. Bend forward deeply to elongate your spine and get your shoulder into the most ideal position. Reach your left arm behind your back and search for your right hand; grasp your left wrist, interlace your fingers, or hold a towel to complete the bind. Align your chest to the centerline of your body so your sternum and pubic bone point forward between your legs. Once your hands are bound, exhale and reach your chin or your forehead to the floor (see fig. 7.13).

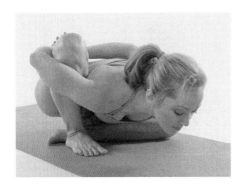

Figure 7.14

Draw your abdomen in and keep your pelvis as level as possible. Keep your sit bones grounded, even as they rise slightly off the ground. If your head does not easily reach the ground, ignore the temptation to round your back forward; instead, elongate and lengthen your torso out of the solid foundation of your pelvis. After five breaths, inhale and straighten your spine; exhale to settle into the pose. Inhale and lift up; exhale and jump back. Repeat the pose on the opposite side.

BENEFITS

Cleanses the liver, kidneys, and abdominal organs
Improves digestion
Opens the hips and shoulders
Deepens the bandhas

MARICHASANA C

Pose Dedicated to Sage Marichi C

Drishti: Parsva (Side)

This pose deeply cleanses your digestive system by twisting your spine and torso. When you use the support of your abdominal and back muscles to facilitate twisting, this cleansing motion is both safe and effective.

Inhale, jump through from Downward-Facing Dog following the last vinyasa in Marichasana B, and begin with both legs outstretched in Dandasana. Bend your right leg and place your right foot flat on the floor near the outside edge of your right hip joint and the heel just in front of the sit bone with a hand's distance between your foot and your left thigh (the same position as in Marichasana A). Keep both sit bones firmly planted on the ground and your pelvis as symmetrically aligned as possible.

Draw your lower belly in and lift your spine out of your pelvis, feeling the energy reach and extend out through the top of your head. On an inhalation, lift your chest and reach from your waist and torso over to the right, while bringing your left arm up and to the right. As you exhale, lean over to the right with your whole torso, twist your spine, and reach your left arm down around your right thigh. Rotate your left shoulder downward while

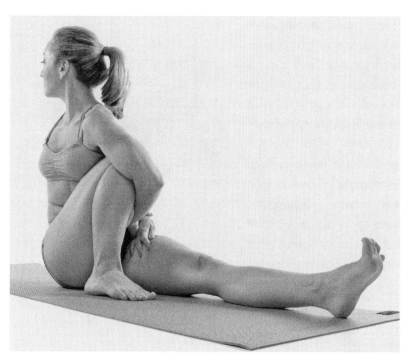

Figure 7.15

engaging the muscles around your shoulder girdle on the left side, including the serratus anterior, deltoid, and lattisimus dorsi. The fingers of your left hand start off pointing toward the ceiling, but as you rotate your left shoulder forward, your left elbow bends naturally, creating a bind around your right shin and knee. Reach the fingers of your left hand toward your upper left thigh. This becomes the receiving hand and should not activate too much once it is in place. As you exhale reach your right hand around your back and allow both hands to make contact above your upper left thigh. Clasp your fingers together or hold your right wrist with your left hand. If you unable to reach your hands, either allow them to float in the air or use a towel to create a bind. Once you have achieved this bind by yourself or with assistance, check to be sure that your pelvis has not shifted from one side to the other and align the back of your pelvis in as straight a line as possible. Check that your lower back is not rounded; it should be lifted and supported up and out of the pelvis (see fig. 7.15).

Eventually this movement is performed as you create space as you jump through on one inhalation and then take the bind and enter the pose on one exhalation. However, take your time if you are a beginner and use your breath to open your body.

Every inhalation creates length and spaciousness in your body, and every exhalation uses that space to bend safely. Every movement is a combination of strength and flexibility. If you are naturally strong, you will need to breathe deeply to get your strength to soften; if you are naturally flexible, you will need to concentrate your mind to be sharp and precise so that your body will strengthen.

In the complete version of this pose, you will feel energy traveling up to the top of your head. Despite this upward motion of energy, be careful not to change the rotation of your left shoulder forward and the position of your torso or you will twist yourself right out of the bind. Keep your shoulder girdle in a position so that your left shoulder rotates downward while the right one opens backward. If you can bind your wrist, then press down into your left thigh with your right fingers. You need to keep your torso as close to your right thigh as possible and lean as much of your body around your right thigh as you can. Also, keep your abdomen drawn in so the purification of your internal organs takes place and your spine is supported. Think about the twisting motion as beginning from just above the pubic bone with the combination of a lean to the side and a twist along the spinal axis. Both sit bones should be on the ground, and your right knee should remain aligned over your right foot. The slight inward rotation of your right hip joint flexes your hip and deepens the pose.

After five breaths come out of the pose on an inhalation. Continue to inhale as you lift up and exhale to jump back, then repeat the pose on the opposite side.

BENEFITS

Cleanses and massages the abdominal organs
Improves digestion
Relieves constipation
Opens the spine and shoulders
Deepens the bandhas
Relieves back pain
Increases energy flow

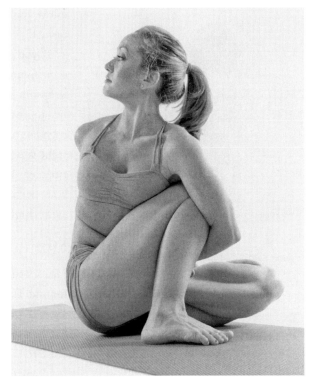

Figure 7.16

MARICHASANA D

Pose Dedicated to Sage Marichi D

Drishti: Parsva (Side)

Marichasana D is one of the most challenging poses in the Ashtanga Yoga series. Considered to be a gateway pose, this movement challenges your ability to rotate your hip joints externally and internally, open your shoulders, twist deeply from your spine, and support your lower back. Full attainment of the pose indicates proficiency in at least half of the Primary Series. To avoid unnecessary injury, surrender your ego and relax your effort in this pose.

Inhale, jump through to a seated position from Downward-Facing Dog following the last vinyasa of Marichasana C, and begin in Dandasana. Take your left leg into half-lotus position as outlined in Ardha Baddha Padma Paschimattanasana. Place the top of your left foot as close to your right hip crease as possible, aligning the heel with your lower belly. If you are unable to perform half-lotus position, take five breaths in your best half-lotus to open your hip joint and focus on external rotation. Modify the half-lotus by simply bending your left knee and tucking your left foot under the top of your right thigh (see fig. 7.17). Continuing either with half-lotus or modification, bend your right knee and plant your right foot flat on the ground so that your foot aligns with the outer edge of your right hip joint. Lean your weight forward so your left knee touches the floor, and

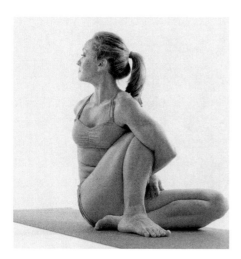

Figure 7.17

allow your right sit bone to rise slightly, if necessary. Even if your right sit bone lifts away from the floor, keep a sense of groundedness in it.

If you feel pain in your left knee, stop here for five breaths and then continue with the easy modification. If you do not feel pain in your knee, keep the half-lotus and hug your right knee to your chest; flex your right hip joint deeply, and draw your abdomen in to support your spine. Holding your torso close to your right leg encourages an internal rotation of the right hip joint that is necessary for deep twisting. Inhale as you lift your rib cage, spine, and torso up and over your right thigh from down inside your pelvis. Reach your whole torso to the right, lifting it fully around your right thigh.

MODIFICATION

Hook your left shoulder around your right lower thigh and knee in the same manner as Marichasana C. Reach and rotate your left shoulder around your right thigh so the elbow bends naturally around your right shin. Rest your left hand on your left leg as it is folded in lotus position. Keep your torso close to your thigh as you reach around your right leg. Avoid pushing too hard with your left arm, and focus on creating space within your pelvis and spine to enter the pose. You may need to put your right hand on the floor behind you to help transfer your weight forward.

Roll your right shoulder blade down your back, transfer your weight forward, and exhale as you clasp your hands together to bind the pose near your left thigh. Once your hands make contact, either interlace your fingers or hold your right wrist with your left hand. When your hands come together, the balance will feel very precarious. Draw your abdomen in and engage your pelvic floor, allowing your weight to pour into your right big toe. Soften your left knee; do not squeeze it or force it down to the floor (see fig. 7.16).

If you cannot bring your hands together, you can either allow them to float toward each other or use a towel or belt to create a bind. Once you have achieved this bind by yourself or with assistance, check to be sure that your pelvis has not shifted too far from one side to the other and align the back of your pelvis in as straight a line as possible. Check that your right foot and left knee are not too far apart or too close together. Be sure that your lower back is not rounded; it should be lifted and supported up and out of your pelvis.

Eventually, this movement is performed as you jump through on one inhalation and then take the bind and enter the pose on one exhalation, as indicated in the vinyasa count appendix. However, take your time if you are a beginner and use your breath to open your body. Do not rush the movement. The healing benefits of this pose come from wringing out your digestive system and torso like a wet towel. Toxins will flood your bloodstream as they release from the rest of your body. Breathe deeply and remain calm.

ADVANCED POSE WITH BOTH SIT BONES DOWN

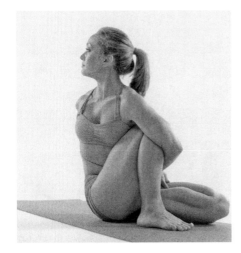

Figure 7.18

Some students can enter the complete pose with both sit bones on the ground, but this is not recommended for beginners or even intermediate students (see fig. 7.18). There are many roadblocks to achieving this pose, but if you practice regularly and relax your effort, you will find your way. Remember to take each movement as a complete step, and do not rush into attempting the bind. Listen to your body and be sure that you have fully integrated each step before moving on to the next. If you feel a sense of panic or restricted breathing, relax into the uncertainty. Over time, you will learn how to breathe into new spaces in your lungs to get a full, deep breath while in this pose.

After five breaths, inhale and lift up; exhale and jump back. Repeat the pose on the opposite side.

BENEFITS

Cleanses and massages the abdominal organs
Improves digestion
Relieves constipation
Opens the spine and shoulders
Deepens the bandhas
Relieves back pain
Increases energy flow

NAVASANA

Boat Pose

Drishti: Padhayoragrai (Toes)

There are two parts to this pose, and both are repeated five times to build strength. The first portion (see fig. 7.19) is typically referred to as Navasana by all the yoga traditions, whereas the second portion (see fig. 7.20) is more commonly referred to as Lolasana (Pendant Pose) in styles other than Ashtanga. Both are repeated, challenging movements that train your core muscles.

Inhale and jump through to a seated position from Downward-Facing Dog following the last vinyasa of Marichasana D. Bend your knees and roll your pelvis under toward the back of your sit bones. Allow the flesh between the sit bones and the tailbone to melt into the floor. Before attempting

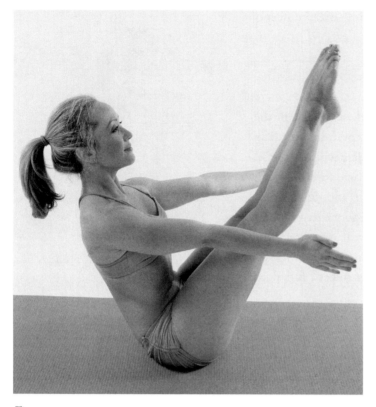

Figure 7.19

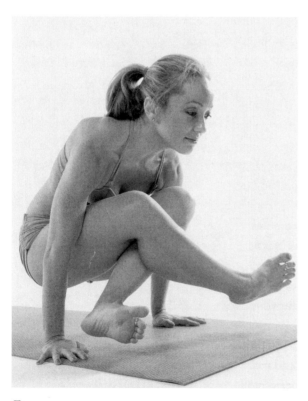

Figure 7.20

to lift your legs off the ground, build a foundation from the inside of your pelvis. Let your sit bones, tailbone, and pubic bone move toward each other while you strongly engage your pelvic floor.

Gently pull in your abdomen, and draw your stomach back toward your spine. Once this inward motion is accomplished, let your stomach draw down so that it feels like you are thrusting your sit bones into the ground from within. Like anchors that hold your body in place, your sit bones and the bottom of your pelvis should feel firmly planted in the ground. Once your foundation is strong, allow your legs to lift and straighten as an extension of this inner awareness. Pull the heads of the femurs deeply into your pelvis. Press your big toes together and engage the inside of your quadriceps to encourage a slight inward rotation. Try not to overuse your hip flexors; instead, lift your lower body with deeper, more internal muscles. Lift your spine out of your pelvis to create length and lift your torso. Ignore the temptation to round your back. Arms are straight and parallel with the floor, shoulders are rolled down your back, and chest is raised.

If you find this pose challenging, you may, for a limited time, bend your knees while lifting your feet off the floor, as long as you are still doing the work of strengthening the interior space of your pelvis. Each time you do Navasana, try to straighten your legs a little more so that your body is at a ninety-degree angle. If you are not able to do this in five repetitions of five breaths each, you can build up to the full version of the pose with regular practice. Do not compromise the work of your pelvis for a higher lift of your legs. After one round of five breaths, move into the second portion of the pose.

The second portion involves lifting your entire body off the ground. You perform this lift in between the five successive Navasana repetitions so that the interior work on your pelvis accelerates in intensity, and it can actually get very strong if you maintain inner awareness. Enter the movement directly from the first part of Navasana; bend your knees into your chest, cross them at the shins as in the photo, and hold them there as tightly as possible. Place your hands on the floor a few inches in front of your pelvis slightly wider than your hips. Engage your upper body, strengthen your shoulder girdle, and keep your abdomen drawn in and your pelvic floor engaged. Lean forward into your arms and lift yourself up. Try not to let your feet touch the floor, but if they do, keep lifting your hips higher, drawing the heads of your femurs into the hip joints, and squeezing your knees into your chest. If you can lift your hips but not your feet, keep practicing and the strength will come. Beginners can try lifting only one foot at a time after they feel solid in lifting the hips while leaning forward into the arms.

Keeping your legs tucked into your body is crucial in the lift section. If your legs are soft, they cannot float when you lean your weight forward into your arms. Practicing Navasana deepens the flexion of the hip joint, and if done with inner awareness of the interior space of your pelvis, it can easily prepare your legs to lift lightly off the ground. After one breath, gently come down and enter the first phase of Navasana again. Repeat five times, then jump directly back as you exhale.

BENEFITS

Relieves constipation
Strengthens the core muscles
Energizes the kidneys, prostate, and thyroid

BHUJAPIDASANA

Shoulder Pressing Pose

Drishti: Nasagrai (Nose)

Bhujapidasana is the first arm balance of the Ashtanga Yoga Primary Series. It combines the external hip rotation and basic strength developed in the vinyasa movements in a challenging yet accessible way. If you have never tried an arm balance before, it will feel like a magical lift off the ground and test your boundaries for what you believe is possible. Start with a relaxed attitude and be willing to put in the work it takes over a long period. Both the pose itself and the traditional entry and exit are demanding. The complete movement requires mental and physical stamina. Do not quit, even if it seems absolutely impossible at first. Surrender to the whole learning and evolutionary process.

From Adho Mukha Svanasana, jump your feet forward and apart so that they are on the outside edges of your hands. Walk your feet even farther forward so they move ahead of your hands. Allow your hip joints to flex and your thighs to separate from your torso and roll forward of your shoulders like in Marichasana A. For an easy setup, bend your arms slightly and step on your hands while keeping the heels of both hands planted firmly on the ground and allowing the thighs to rest on the shelf of the upper

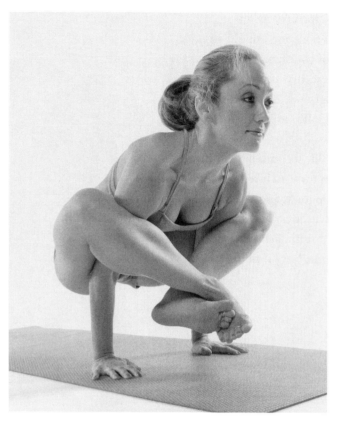

Figure 7.21

arms. If you find this challenging, stop here and work on this movement for five breaths, then jump back. If you are able to continue, lower your hips slightly while keeping your thighs above your elbows and engage your shoulder girdle for upper body support. Grip your fingertips slightly into the floor, feel the strength of your body, and engage the pelvic floor. Once you feel stable here, bend your knees and walk your feet closer together in front of your hands until the big toes touch. Keep your feet on the floor as you inch them toward each other; the weight of your body stays supported by your hands and core strength. If you find this difficult, stay here for five breaths and then jump back.

Continuing the motion, cross your right foot over your left, flex them firmly around each other, and hold that position. Once you feel stable, press into your arms, lean forward slightly, and lift your feet off the floor in a flexed position without falling backward (see fig. 7.21). Thrust firmly into your hands, opening your collarbones, and drawing your shoulder blades down your back; support your body with a firm lift from your abdomen. If you are new to the pose, stay here for five breaths and keep your weight away from the floor. Send your chest forward without arching your back, lift your pelvis, and press firmly down into your hands.

If you can balance in the preliminary movement, exhale and bring the top of your head down to the floor while maintaining the support in your hands and arms. Walk your feet through the space between your hands, point your toes, and lift your feet completely off the floor while keeping your ankles crossed (see fig. 7.22). If you can maintain balance throughout the movement, keep your feet floating while you bend your arms and lift your feet between your hands.

Advanced students who can flow through these movements easily can jump directly into the first portion of the pose, where you cross your feet and balance on your hands, in one breath. If you are this advanced, you should reach your chin and not the top of your head to the floor, keeping your feet off the ground for the whole movement. This is the complete version of the pose (see fig. 7.23).

Whether you have the top of your head or your chin on the floor, hold the pose for five breaths, then lift your head off the ground and bring your feet back to the front of your hands. Repeat whichever movement you used to get your feet behind your hands, walking on the floor or floating them back. When you lift your head, think about sending your chest forward while pressing firmly into your arms. You ideally exit a pose with same level of integrity as when you entered it. Be careful not to let too much weight rest in your hips or else you will fall backward. If that happens, just pick yourself up and try again. Give yourself at least three tries every day, but no more.

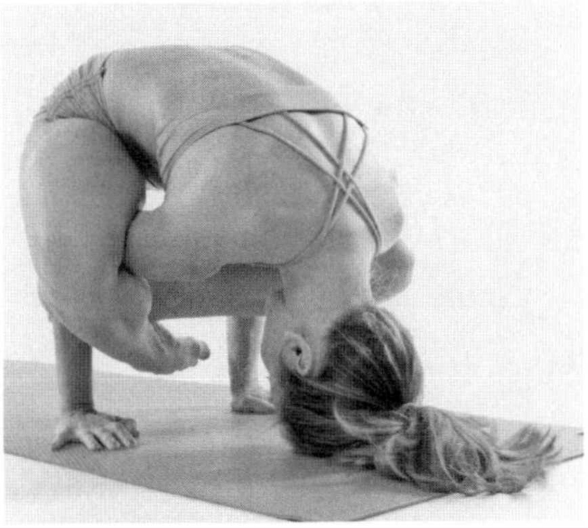

Jumping back from this pose requires endurance and stamina of the mind and body. First, find your balance again in the preparation stage where your feet are crossed and you are balancing on your arms. Lean to your right and bring your left leg around so that the left knee is bent and sits as close to the left armpit as possible. Then lean to the left and bring your right leg around to a similar position. This transition passes through a posture called Bakasana (Crow Pose). Bend both of your arms and exhale to jump back. Originate the movement from your core and breathe deeply. Take as many breaths as you need to complete the movement; do not rush. Do not worry about attaining a perfect transition, just lean your chest forward and press your arms to jump back.

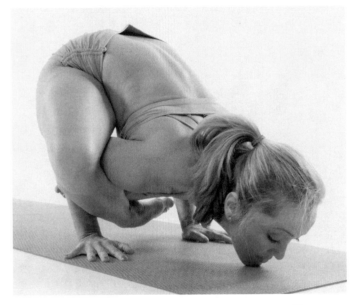

Figure 7.22

If you are an advanced student, you will be able to bring both feet around your arms at the same time by leaning your chest forward and lifting your pelvis in equal measure up and forward over your arms. Once in Bakasana position, lean your body weight farther forward while bending your arms slightly to initiate the jump back. There will be a strong temptation to put your feet down before jumping back. Breathe deeply and keep your body lifted with the strength of your shoulder girdle and your core muscles. Let the interior space of your body do the work in the pose as much as possible. Exhale as you jump back to Chaturanga Dandasana.

Figure 7.23

BENEFITS

Improves balance
Strengthens the core, arms, shoulders, and wrists
Purifies the abdominal organs
Builds self-confidence

KURMASANA/SUPTA KURMASANA

Tortoise Pose/Sleeping Tortoise Pose

Drishti: Nasagrai (Nose)

These two poses form one of the great gateway poses of the Ashtanga Yoga Primary Series, and they test the strength, stability, and openness of both

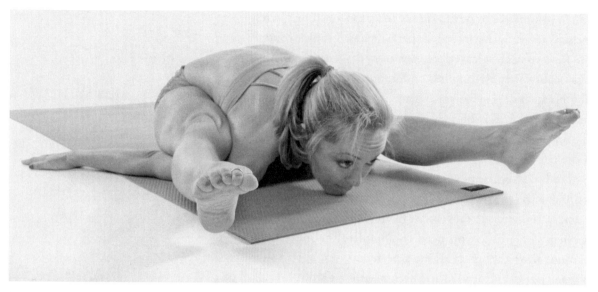

Figure 7.24

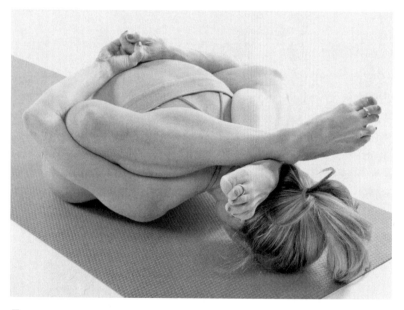

Figure 7.25

body and mind. This movement asks you to have a good understanding of the bandhas, hip rotation, and elongation of the back muscles. The challenge of moving deeply into the pelvis and the hip joints here may be rather intense. Proceed slowly, giving your body the time and space it needs to open.

From Adho Mukha Svanasana, jump or step your feet around your hands, walking them as far forward as you can so that your thighs hug your shoulders and your torso fits between your thighs as much as possible. Bend your elbows, allow your hips to sink to the ground, then slide your hands out to the side, palms facing downward. You might feel like letting your hips hit the ground with a clunk, but try to control the movement as much as possible. (More proficient students will be able to jump directly into position, with the thighs resting on the upper arms and balancing above the ground before allowing the hips to sink.) Once your hips and pelvis are on the ground, extend your legs out from your hips and straighten your legs and knees. Ignore the temptation to let your legs widen by squeezing your thighs as close to your shoulders as possible. Flatten your back by elongating your spine and torso. Reach your heart and the center of your chest toward the floor and open your collarbones by pressing your shoulders into your thighs to prevent any compression around the front of your chest. Roll your shoulder blades down your back while engaging your shoulder girdle for both stability and openness through your chest, hips, and back.

If you can, engage your legs until they are totally straight and your heels lift off the ground. To lift your legs higher, pull the head of each femur deeper into its hip socket and activate your pelvic floor. Engage the insides of your knees and press your chin into the ground while lifting your hips, thereby creating deeper flexion of the hip joints and space to slide your torso farther back between your thighs. Breathe deeply through your whole body, but don't breathe too much into your abdomen. Try to soften and relax your hip joints while allowing energy to flow freely throughout the interior space of your pelvis. Stay in Kurmasana for five breaths (see fig. 7.24).

Moving into Supta Kurmasana (see fig. 7.25) requires that you rotate your hip joints externally while keeping the elongation in your back muscles and the openness in your shoulder girdle. Begin by turning your knees out to the sides and slide your arms even farther back under your thighs; bending your arms back will cause your shoulders to rotate. If possible, bring your feet as close together as possible. Rotate your shoulders downward and elongate the joints so that your hands reach up around the lower portion of your back. See if you can interlock your fingers or hold your wrist as you exhale. You can hold a towel if your hands won't touch. If you are practicing with a teacher, this is the place to wait for an adjustment to help take you deeper.

Once your hands are interlocked, cross your right ankle over the left in front of your head, or bring your feet as close together as possible. More advanced students will find that sitting up and placing both legs behind the head is a better option for going deeper into the pose. If you are attempting the more advanced method, you should master crossing your ankles on the floor or seek the assistance of a teacher first. Be careful to locate the external rotation in your hip joints. If you feel pressure on your knees while moving into the beginner or advanced version, back off.

Having both legs behind your head increases the upward flow of energy along your spine and demands a high degree of openness in your pelvis and hip joints. It also requires stability deep within the body. After holding with your ankles crossed for five breaths, inhale as you lift directly off the ground, keeping your legs crossed behind your head (see fig. 7.26). To lift up while maintaining the full posture, spread your arms slightly wider than shoulder width apart when lifting up from the floor. Engage your deltoids and your shoulder girdle while pressing your neck back into your legs. Begin looking up as you press your arms into the ground with the same power cultivated

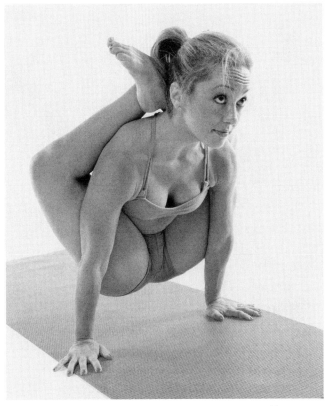

Figure 7.26

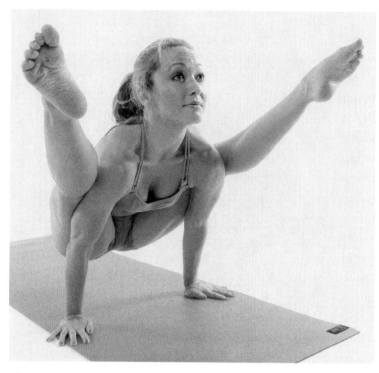

Figure 7.27

in the vinyasas and in Navasana. Release your feet, coming into Tittibhasana or Firefly Pose (see fig 7.27). Although this is a full posture in the Intermediate Series, you pass through it only in transition, so do not worry too much about perfecting it. Just move through the pose as best as possible. Exhale as you take back your legs to Bakasana pose (see fig 7.28) in the same manner as in Bujapidasana. In full Bakasana pose the knees are placed directly into the armpits, but in the Primary Series, this pose is a transition; just pass through it to the best of your ability. The key lesson of this transition is to move through the best possible version of the challenging poses while keeping your feet off the ground. Do not stop to set up for these poses; just flow through them. After you reach Bakasana, exhale as you jump back to Chaturanga Dandasana.

The entire movement will challenge your endurance and stamina. This energetic pose deeply heals past emotional hurt, particularly around the hip joints, and increases inner awareness of the body. If you cannot perform this pose with ease in your daily practice, I advise stopping here before moving on. Skip the remaining seated poses and proceed to the backbending section.

Benefits

Opens the hips and the energy channels around the hips
Strengthens the shoulders
Improves digestion
Treats depression, anxiety, and anger
Builds endurance

Garbha Pindasana

Womb Embryo Pose

Drishti: Nasagrai (Nose)

This is the first full lotus position of the Primary Series. You may find it strange that it comes after you've put your legs behind your head, but this pose comprises far more than merely sitting in lotus position. It involves having enough relaxed, dynamic control of the position to generate movement within the lotus. Additionally, since the knees are fully bent, it requires the full rotation of the hip joints along with complete relaxation of the lower back and interior space of the pelvis. So in some ways this is a more demanding movement than Supta Kurmasana.

Start out by following the healthy external rotation techniques outlined for Ardha Baddha Padma Paschimat-tanasana. If you can do half-lotus comfortably, which should be possible if you can perform all the preceding poses in the Primary Series with relative ease, then begin rotating the right leg externally, making sure your knee joint is closed and the knee points out to the side. Lift your right knee slightly as you bring your left foot under your right shin to move into seated half-lotus position. Once you feel comfortable here, take your left knee out to the side even more while keeping your knee joints closed. Allow your right knee to float toward the ground, but do not push it there. Gently lift your left foot over your right shin, aiming the top of the foot toward your right hip crease. Be careful not to let your right foot slip off as you direct your left foot into position. Ideally, both heels will align on the outside edges of your navel so that when you fold your lotus in toward your body, your heels will press into the interior space of your pelvis.

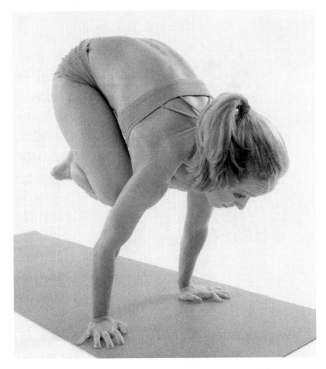

Figure 7.28

If you feel comfortable in lotus position and are able to relax completely, then you can move further into the full expression of the pose. If you find the full lotus position challenging, do not attempt to force your way into the pose. You can proceed by continuing from half-lotus pose after reaching your maximum capacity or proceed directly to backbends, skipping the remainder of the seated poses.

Continuing with the pose, draw your legs into your chest. If you are working with half-lotus, wrap both of your arms around your thighs and hold your bottom foot to support it underneath. If you are working with full lotus position, aim your hands through the small holes between your upper calf and your thigh. If your hands get stuck, roll up your pants (or wear shorts) and spray yourself with water to make your skin more slippery. Next, cup your hands and aim them, fingers first, toward the center, through the seemingly imperceptible holes and twist your arms from your fingers to your elbows

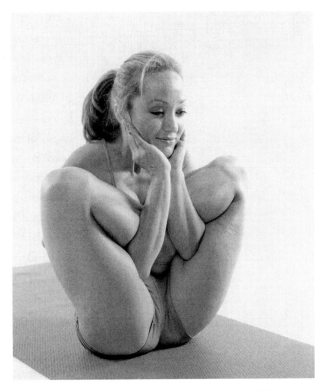

Figure 7.29

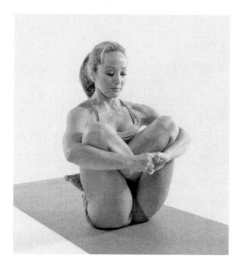

Figure 7.30

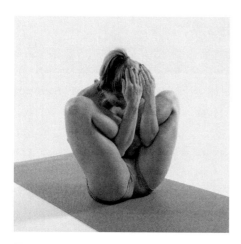

Figure 7.31

like corkscrews. Once you get as far as your elbows, bend your arms, continue twisting, and follow the spiraling motion to support the rotation of your arms through your legs.

You may find it easier to start off with your right arm and get it all the way through. Then once the left arm gets in a little more than halfway, you can use your right hand to grip the left and pull it through. Finally, bend your elbows deeply, reach your hands to your ears, and gaze at the tip of your nose (see fig. 7.29). Be careful not to squeeze your knees while you are trying to wiggle your arms through your legs. If you can get into lotus position but cannot reach your hands through, then merely hold your lotus into the chest and bind your hands together around your legs.

Once you find your balance, use your bandhas to ground your pelvis firmly while creating space around your hip joints to rotate outward even farther. Beginners will find that merely holding the lotus or half-lotus position into the body while grabbing the thighs really challenges their sense of balance (see fig. 7.30). Apply the same grounding principles as you used in Navasana. The strength you developed inside your pelvis establishes the awareness you need to roll over your spine in the next step of this and many other poses in the remainder of the series.

Once you are able to take five breaths in this balancing position, you are ready to begin rolling up and down on the outside of your spine, exhaling as you go back and inhaling as you come up. To prepare, hold your head with your hands and roll down along the outer portion of your right back muscles and up along the outer portion of your left back muscles, keeping the movement as close to your spine as possible without putting pressure on the vertebrae (see fig. 7.31). The first time you try this, you may want to go up and down in the same position just to get used to the movement. If you have a thin yoga mat, place a towel under your spine for the initial stages of rolling. Once you get proficient at the movement, you will not need any additional padding.

After you are able to easily roll up and down five times in the same position, you can try rolling to the right in a circle, turning very slightly on each backward and forward movement. Draw your abdomen in and direct your movement based on your center of gravity. Use your pelvis as the steering wheel for your body and avoid using your hands to direct the movement. Relax your shoulders and allow your inner strength to control the whole movement. Do not give up if you fall off to the side; use your pelvis to return to your back and begin again, initiating the movement with the breath so that you exhale down and inhale up while turning slightly. Although traditionally, you get five rolls to return to your starting point, take as many as you need while you are learning. Continue immediately into the next pose with no vinyasa.

BENEFITS

Builds the bandhas, core strength, and awareness of the
    central axis
Improves digestion
Increases balance
Strengthens the entire body

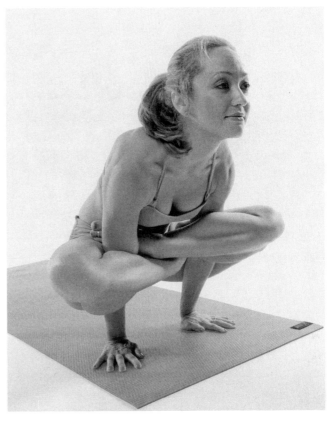

Figure 7.32

KUKKUTASANA

Cock Pose

Drishti: Nasagrai (Nose)

Enter this pose directly from Garbha Pindasana. Inhale
after you return to center and roll all the way up to a seated
position. If you are in full lotus and your arms are through
your legs, you will need to allow your legs to slide down
slightly so they are closer to the ground and your wrists. If
you are in either half-lotus or full lotus without your arms
through your legs, then place your hands in the same position as they were in the lift-up between Navasana counts.
Whichever version you are using, lean your body weight forward into your
hands and press the base of the fingers, fingertips, and heel of each hand
firmly into the ground. Pull in your lower belly, squeeze your lower ribs
toward each other, engage your legs, and draw your shoulder blades down
your back. Be careful not to lean so far forward that you fall. Find the perfect balance between too much and too little effort (see fig. 7.32).

Draw your knees as far into your chest as possible and breathe deeply.
Allow your strength to come from your whole body. After five deep breaths,
release the pose, gently releasing your hands and removing your arms from
between your thighs but keeping the lotus position if you can. More advanced students can jump back directly from lotus position. Beginners
can release their version of lotus or half-lotus and then jump back from a
simple cross-legged position. Remember to inhale as you lift up and exhale
to jump back to Chaturanga Dandasana.

BENEFITS

Builds the bandhas, core strength, and awareness of the central axis
Improves digestion
Increases balance
Strengthens the entire body
Increases self-confidence

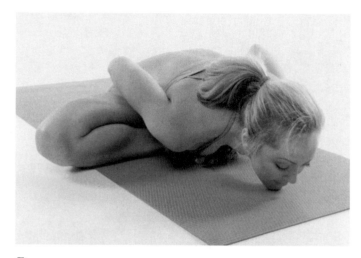

Figure 7.33

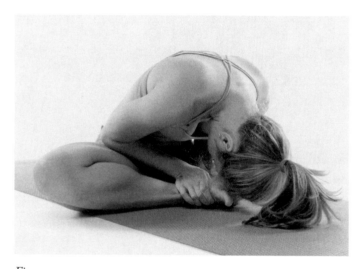

Figure 7.34

BADDHA KONASANA A AND B

Bound Angle Pose A and B

Drishti: Nasagrai (Nose)

This pose involves an external rotation of both hip joints and a full bend in the knees, doubling the flexibility required in Janu Sirsasana A. Be careful from the beginning not to force yourself into the pose and damage your knees. Be patient and allow the movement to come from your hip joints and a release of your inner thighs.

Inhale and jump through to a seated position from Downward-Facing Dog. Begin by drawing the soles of your feet together. Press the outer edges of both feet together and, holding your feet at the base of the big toe mound in the ball of each foot, use your hands to actively turn the soles of your feet toward the ceiling. Keep the outside edges of your feet by the little toes together so that the bases of the little toes and the outside of the heels maintain contact. Keep pressing your heels together and keep your legs active. Your knees should point out to the side and bend as deeply as possible. Keep the knee joints closed while thrusting your feet into each other to help protect your knees while your hips and thighs open. If this pose is new to you, expect to feel a steady burning sensation along your inner thighs and around your hip joints closest to the pelvis.

Breathe deeply, and draw your pelvic floor and abdomen in. Make sure your spine is straight.

Once you have established your foundation in your legs, begin applying the safe forward bend technique used throughout the Primary Series to reach your chest and chin toward the floor and send your pubic bone back as you exhale. Keep your back straight for the first version of the pose, lengthening and elongating your back muscles, and ignore the temptation to round your back to get closer to the floor (see fig. 7.33). Gravity needs time to soften your inner thighs, so give this pose more than the usual five breaths if necessary to reach maximum flexibility. Get your pelvis as close to your feet as possible when you fold forward. After at least five breaths, inhale back to an upright straight spine and then exhale to round your back for the second version.

Draw your abdomen in strongly and support your spine's movement into deeper flexion to enter Baddha Konasana B (see fig. 7.34). Round your back and aim the top of your head at your insteps. Be careful not to compress your spine; use the spaciousness created by your strong inner work to enter the pose safely and easily. Stay in it for five breaths.

My teacher would recommend that students who felt very tight in their hips hold this pose for up to fifty breaths. But if you feel a burning or pinching sensation in your knees, that is a sign to back off, not to go deeper. The pain may lessen if you place a towel, block, or bolster under each knee. If, however, you feel intense sensations in your ankles, back muscles, hip joints, or inner thighs, that is a sign that the pose is targeting the intended areas. Continue on with caution, care, and love.

Return to a straight spine on an inhalation. Exhale and hold the pose (see fig. 7.35). Then inhale to lift up; exhale to jump back.

Benefits

Cleanses the kidneys, bladder, prostate, ovaries, and
    other abdominal organs
Opens the kidney meridian
Improves circulation
Stretches the inner thighs, groin, and hips
Treats fatigue
Aids in childbirth

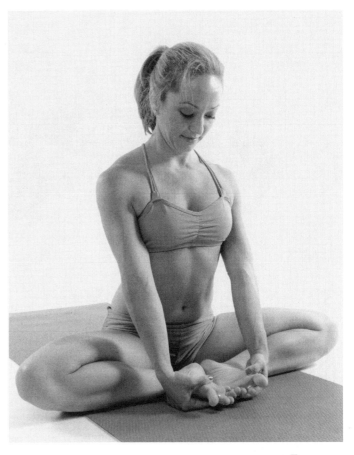

Figure 7.35

Upavistha Konasana

Wide-Angle Seated Forward Bend

Drishti: Nasagrai (Nose) and Urdhva (Up to the Sky)

Inhale, and jump through to a seated position from Downward-Facing Dog following the last vinyasa in Baddha Konasana. Spread your legs wide apart and hold on to the outside edge of each foot. Your legs should be as far apart as the width of your shoulder girdle allows. There is no need to attempt a full straddle here, as the purpose of this pose is more on releasing your back forward and deepening the rotation of your hip joints in relation to your torso. Once your legs are spread and you are holding your feet, engage your arms just enough to guide your shoulder blades down your back. Do not pull too hard or you may overstretch your inner thigh and hamstring.

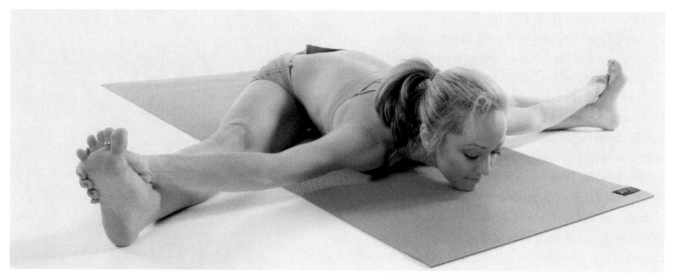

Figure 7.36

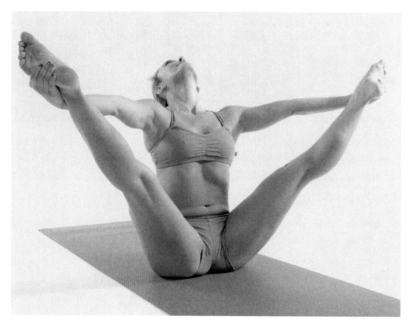

Figure 7.37

Moving gently from the waist, draw your lower belly in and let gravity help your torso slide down between your thighs to enter the pose (see fig. 7.36). Draw your trochanters (the upper portion of the thighbone near the pelvis) back to ground your pelvis and prevent your sit bones from rising off the floor. Engage your quadriceps and send energy out through the base of each big toe while pulling the heads of your thighbones into your pelvis. Keep the feet flexed. Be careful not to pooch your belly out. For the first segment of this pose, it is crucial that you relax your effort and be gentle with your body. If you cannot reach your chin to the floor, place the top of your head on the floor. If this is impossible while maintaining a relatively straight spine, breathe patiently and soon it will be possible. Opening your inner thighs releases a key meridian for kidney and sugar balance in the body. Stay in this position for at least five breaths.

For the second portion of the pose, lean back so your pelvis is in the same position as it was in Navasana, with your abdomen drawn in and your pelvic floor engaged. Inhale as you let go of your feet, lift your legs with either straight or bent knees, and again grip the outsides of your feet near the little toes in a balancing position (see fig 7.37). Engage your legs fully and reach them outward from the base of each big toe; point your feet and counterbalance by drawing the head of each femur deeper into its hip socket. Lift your spine up and out of your pelvis to create the hint of a spinal extension and look up while raising the sternum. Make sure your pelvis is planted firmly on the ground and supported by your inner body. To make the transition out of intense forward bends into backbends, which comes at the end of the practice, you must be able to release your spine and gently encourage extension. This pose goes from a forward bend that is supported on the floor to a balance that encourages extension and strengthens your back muscles. Balance here for five breaths. Take your hands to the floor. Inhale and lift up; exhale and jump back to Chaturanga Dandasana.

BENEFITS

Cleanses the kidneys, bladder, prostate, ovaries, and
　　other abdominal organs
Opens the kidney meridian
Improves circulation
Stretches the inner thighs, groin, and hips
Treats fatigue

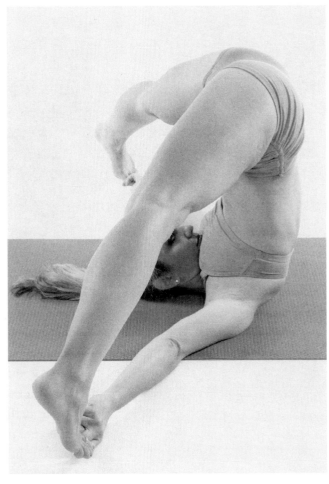

Figure 7.38

SUPTA KONASANA

Reclining Angle Pose

Drishti: Nasagrai (Nose)

Inhale and jump through to a seated position from Downward-Facing Dog after the last vinyasa from Upavistha Konasana. Exhale as you lie flat on your back. Inhale and lift your legs over the top of your head so that you roll all the way onto your shoulders. Touch your toes to the floor and spread your legs as wide apart as the length of your arms permits. Grasp your big toes firmly and flex your feet while taking the majority of your weight on your shoulders and your big toes. Leave enough space for at least a finger under the arch of your neck when you enter the pose fully (see fig. 7.38). Lift your spine out of your pelvis so that your back muscles support and lift your body. Keep your hips neatly stacked over your shoulders. Ignore the temptation to collapse your back into a rounded position. Draw your lower belly in and lift with your body's own strength. This pose prepares you for inverted poses like Salamba Sarvangasana (Shoulderstand) that come in the finishing sequence and strengthens your back for backbends.

After five breaths, inhale and roll your spine slowly up through a very brief balance and exhale softly as you land on the ground. Keep your legs

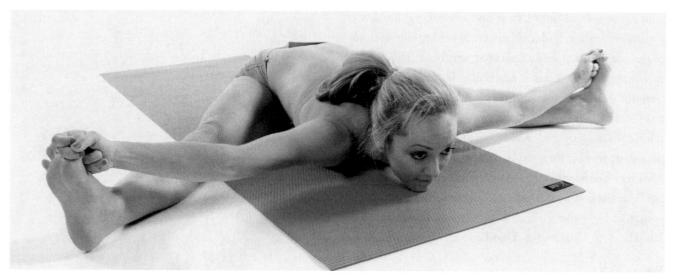

Figure 7.39

straight throughout the movement. Do not hold the balance point; just pause long enough so that you can control the landing. When lowering down, try to land gently by reaching the calf muscles into the floor first and pulling back on your big toes with your fingers. Lower your feet, chest, and chin all the way down to the floor (see fig. 7.39). Just as in the previous pose, do not push when folding forward; simply relax into the movement. After your head and feet touch down, immediately inhale and lift your head while holding on to your toes, exhale and settle into the pose. Inhale and lift up; exhale and jump back.

BENEFITS

Cleanses the kidneys, bladder, prostate, ovaries, and other abdominal
    organs
Opens the kidney meridian
Improves circulation
Stretches the inner thighs, groin, and hips
Treats fatigue
Increases awareness of the body's center of gravity and the bandhas

SUPTA PADANGUSTHASANA

Reclining Big Toe Pose

Drishti: Nasagrai (Nose) and Parsva (Side)

Inhale and jump through to a seated position from Downward-Facing Dog after the last vinyasa of Supta Konasana. Exhale as you lie flat on your back.

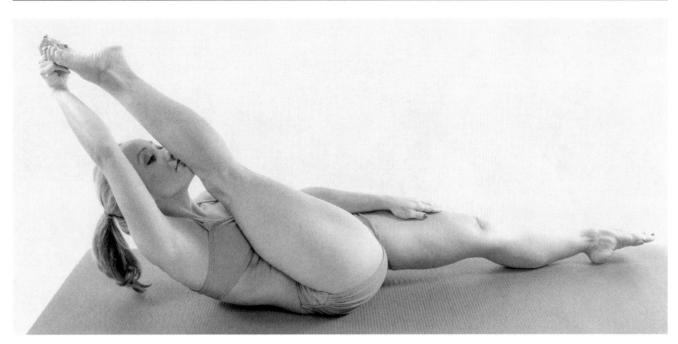

Figure 7.40

Point your toes, press your heels into the ground, and place both hands on top of your thighs. Inhale as you lift your right leg into the air and hold on to your right big toe with your right hand, keeping your left hand firmly on your left thigh. Press your left heel into the ground and stabilize your pelvis by strongly drawing in your abdomen. As you exhale, lift your torso up to meet your right leg. Even if you are flexible enough to place your right foot on the floor by your ear, keep your right leg elevated and reach up with the strength of your body to meet your leg. This pose is not meant purely to increase flexibility but also to build strength. Feel your back and core muscles working to lift your torso while drawing in your lower belly to support that lift. Reach your chin toward your shin and lift strongly (see fig. 7.40). Flexible students should pay careful attention to lifting up into the core strength of the pose. Less flexible students may need to bend their knees to reach the toe and should focus on keeping both legs as straight as possible. After five breaths, inhale and lower your head back to the ground.

Exhale as you extend your right leg out to the side, while maintaining pressure on your left leg with your left hand. Look over your left shoulder. Rotate your right hip joint externally to take your leg fully out to the side (see fig. 7.41). Ignore the temptation to lift your hips off the ground so you can lower your right foot all the way. Instead, allow gravity to do the work for you and concentrate your efforts on keeping your hips stable and lengthening your inner right thigh. Make sure your left leg is stable and firm as your foundation. Pressing the pelvis firmly into the ground will help the hip joints relax. Keep the right foot pointed.

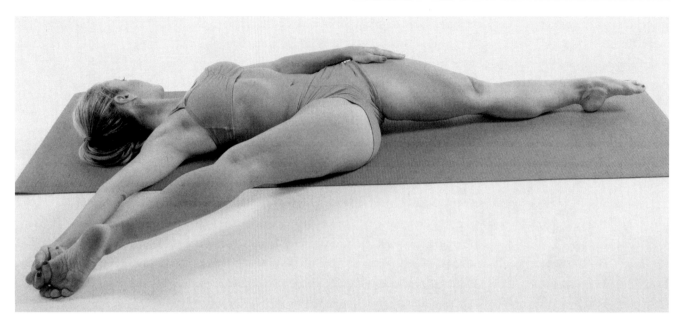

Figure 7.41

After five breaths, inhale and return your right leg to the center position. Exhale, lift up, and touch your chin to your right shin again. Inhale as you put your head down; exhale as you lower your leg. Repeat the sequence on the opposite side. Finally, inhale and roll backward into Chakrasana (Wheel Pose). For a complete explanation of this vinyasa, refer to Chapter 10.

BENEFITS

Strengthens the core muscles
Stretches the hamstrings
Steadies the mind
Stimulates the prostate

UBHAYA PADANGUSTHASANA

Two-Foot Pose

Drishti: Urdhva (Up to the Sky)

Inhale and jump through to a seated position from Downward-Facing Dog after the last vinyasa in Supta Padangusthasana. Exhale as you lie flat on your back. Inhale as you lift your feet over your head and roll onto your shoulders (see fig. 7.43). Clasp your big toes firmly and exhale. Roll forward again one vertebra at a time, keeping your abdomen drawn in. Come up to a balancing position as you inhale to enter the pose fully (see fig. 7.42). If you are proficient at forward bends, keep your legs and arms straight as you roll up. If you are a beginner, you might find it necessary to roll up with bent knees and then enter the full pose once you find the balance in your pelvis. Concentrate your locus of control deep within the center of your body. Ground your pelvis in the floor just as you did in Navasana, lift your spine out of your pelvis, and look up. Lift your sternum to the ceiling and spine away from the pelvis.

This pose teaches you how to maintain full control over each vertebra. By performing the movement, you will develop the inner awareness you need to extend your spine safely. You will also learn how to move from your center of gravity and direct your pelvis with its own inner strength. Do not try to hold the pose with arm strength. Instead, let your arms be relatively free while your shoulders roll down your back. Reach out through the soles of your feet and the base of the big toe. Let each distinct body part be responsible for its own movement. Your spine lifts itself, your legs remain engaged and rotate inward, while you gaze up. Pull the head of each

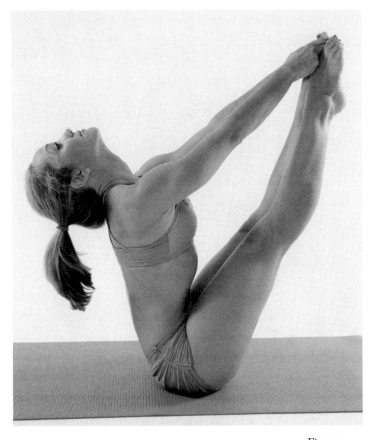

Figure 7.42

femur deeper into its hip socket to ground your pelvis and lift your legs more easily. Press the bases of your big toes together to encourage a slight inward rotation. Point your toes fully. After five breaths, take your hands to the floor and inhale to lift up; exhale and jump back.

BENEFITS

Improves digestion
Stretches the hamstrings
Builds the bandhas, core strength, and awareness of the central axis
Cleanses the internal organs

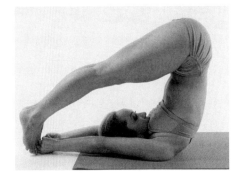

Figure 7.43

URDHVA MUKHA PASCHIMATTANASANA

Upward-Facing Intense Stretch

Drishti: Padhayoragrai (Toes)

Inhale and jump through to a seated position from Downward-Facing Dog following the last vinyasa of the previous pose. Exhale as you lie flat on your back. Inhale as you lift your feet over your head and roll onto your shoulders as in the previous pose (see fig. 7.45). Hold the outside edges

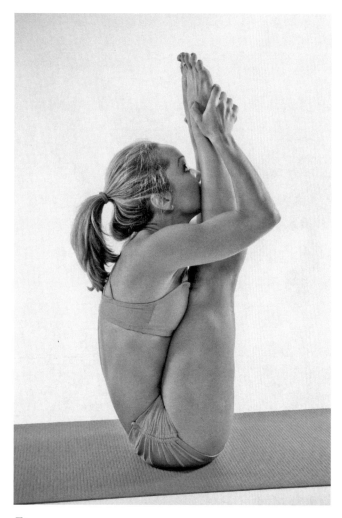

Figure 7.44

of your feet near the heels rather than the big toes. Exhale firmly as you grasp your feet, rolling back so that your weight presses into the pads of your toes to develop momentum so you can push off as you go back. Inhale as you roll up vertebra by vertebra, slowly controlling the movement and coming to a balancing pose with your arms and legs straight (see fig. 7.46). If you feel yourself falling backward, either bend your knees into your chest to roll up or use your toes to pull the weight of your body forward while grounding your hips to roll up with straight legs.

Point your toes as you ground the pelvis with the inner work of the bandhas. Lift your spine out of this solid foundation. Use the strength in your arms to pull your thighs down into the ground and the heads of the femurs deeper into the pelvis. Exhale as you fold forward, bend your arms bringing your chest toward your thighs and your chin toward your shins to enter the pose fully (see fig. 7.44). Look up at your toes. Allow your shoulder blades to roll down your back and increase the sense of grounding in your pelvis. Be conscious of keeping spaciousness around your neck. Let your core muscles rather than your arms do the work of the pose. Let your sit bones melt into the floor and strongly draw your abdomen in. Feel your lower ribs drawing toward the centerline of the body. Be conscious of the three components of the healthy forward bend.

Hold the full pose for five breaths, then inhale as you straighten your arms and look up; exhale as you balance in this position. Place your hands on the floor slightly in front of your pelvis. Inhale and lift up; exhale and jump back.

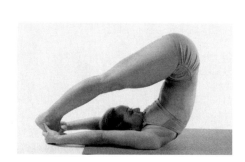

Figure 7.45

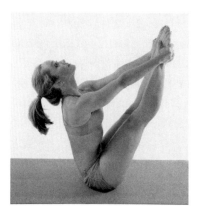

Figure 7.46

BENEFITS

Improves digestion
Stretches the hamstrings
Builds the bandhas, core strength,
    and awareness of the central axis
Cleanses the internal organs

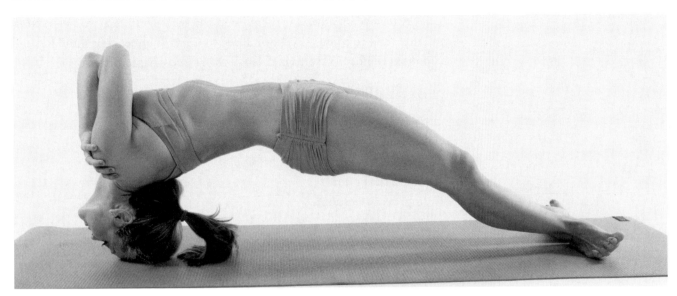

Figure 7.47

SETU BANDHASANA

Spinal Lift Bridge Pose

Drishti: Broomadhya (Eyebrow center)

Inhale and jump through to a seated position. Exhale as you lie flat on your back. Bend your knees, placing your heels together and your toes apart so the toes point outward and the outside edge of each foot by the base of the little toe rests on the floor. Arch your back, placing the top of your head on the floor, and lift your spine completely off the ground (see fig. 7.48); your hips remain on the floor. Cross your arms over each other so that each hand holds the opposite shoulder. As you inhale, lift your hips by sending your body weight into your legs and up to the top of your head to enter the pose fully (see fig. 7.47). Engage your quadriceps and rotate your legs externally to help them straighten. Send your pelvis and tailbone forward; keep your abdomen drawn in. Lift your spine vertebra by vertebra, and engage and elongate your back muscles. Try not to settle your weight in your neck. Open your upper back and lift your sternum. Once you feel stable in the pose, if possible point your toes fully.

This pose prepares your body for backbends by opening the spine, creating strength throughout your erector spinae muscles, and solidifying the sense of foundation and direction in your legs.

You will probably feel an uncomfortable sensation in your neck; if so, you may want to use your hands for support, placing them under your shoulders as you lift your hips off the ground. Gradually lessen your dependence on this support, because the strengthening of the neck plays a crucial role in more advanced poses. As your neck, back, and legs get stronger in this pose, the uncomfortable feeling in the neck will dissipate.

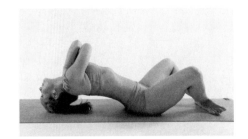

Figure 7.48

After five breaths, exit the pose in the same manner as you entered it, and exhale to come fully down. Place your hands under your shoulders and inhale, rolling backward into Chakrasana (see Chapter 10).

BENEFITS

Stretches and strengthens the neck and back
Lifts energy up the spine
Treats fear, anxiety, and depression
Calms the brain
Improves digestion

8

Backbends: Open Your Heart

WHEN YOU PRACTICE YOGA, YOU SPEND HOURS DELVING into your inner world. The best yoga practitioners are scientists of the spiritual world who search for the highest truths. As you enter this sacred domain, one of the first major challenges you will meet is the test of your emotionality. The poses that most often crack open the Pandora's box of sleeping emotions are backbends.

Emotions have a reality and a life that can sometimes seem larger than you are. When anger or sadness sets in, a biochemical reality changes your heart rate, hormonal balance, and level of muscular tension. Emotions change the chemical balance of your brain and your body. You think differently when you feel angry, sad, anxious, depressed, happy, or in love. Your emotions play a huge role in your overall state of being and color your world with their many hues. Some portion of your life will be spent trying to contain your emotions, reacting to them, or acting on them.

When I first started a daily Mysore-style Ashtanga Yoga practice, my emotions took me for a roller-coaster ride. Not only did I become more aware of my own sensitivity, but the yoga practice unearthed a new heightened awareness of the power and scope of what I was feeling. For example, backbends often brought up sadness that I would otherwise have avoided. I could escape the underlying reality of my feelings for most of the day, but when I opened my spine, I had no place left to hide. Sometimes there would be no physical pain, but the tears came anyway. The overwhelming sense of sadness that releases after deep backbends can feel like the tears of a thousand lifetimes, but you never have to know where the sadness comes from; you just want to observe it and experience it.

The sadness hidden within layers of the emotional body rises to the surface through the tool of asana. The premise of emotional healing through deepening yoga poses is based on the idea that by freeing up and inhabiting every inch of space in your physical and inner body, the light of your awareness unlocks and heals old, stuck emotions and patterns. It is hard to explain, but after a deep backbend, you literally see the world differently because you inhabit your own body with a different consciousness. It was through the emotional journey of the body that I became explicitly conscious of the repercussions of my actions, in tune with the depth of my own feelings, and more clear about everything. I attribute much of my own evolution to the higher insight gained through daily yoga practice.

The particular revelations that followed deep spinal movements were usually associated with releasing, surrendering, letting go. One of the stated purposes of the deep twisting and bending motions in yoga is literally to stir up sleeping areas of the body and the emotions. Backbending did and still does that for me.

In the world of yoga, the body is not separate from the mind. The body can be understood to exist in an energy field that contains your physicality, your thoughts, your emotions, and your spirit. It is within that realm that the yoga poses work. By manipulating your body into pretzel-like positions that defy the master key of logic, you ask your body to go places it has never been before. In doing so, you simultaneously ask your mind to go places it has never been as well. When you act, think, feel, speak, and live from a particular paradigm, it has a lasting impact on your body. Your habitual pose is nothing more than the sum total of your thoughts about yourself written on the canvas of your physical form. Think negative thoughts about yourself and others, and you will see the results in your body over time. Luckily, the magic of yoga practice is that it effects transformation by asking you to move your body in new ways over a long period of time. When you do, your mind, being deeply connected to your body's movement pattern, changes. As you learn to access dormant muscles, tissues, bones, and spaces in your body, you simultaneously learn to access dormant thoughts, emotions, feelings, power, and success.

Backbends are perhaps the greatest teachers available. To get the full benefit from backbends, it is imperative that you think of the movements as coming from more than just "the back." They involve every muscle in your body, including your toes, legs, spine, diaphragm, shoulders, and head. In traditional Urdhva Danurasana (Lifted Bow Pose), the foundation of the backbend is the strength of your legs. Openness along the front of your hip joints (where the thighbones insert into the pelvis) allows your pelvis to tilt forward and move over your legs and the iliac crests to move forward. Each vertebra lifts and extends with the support of your core and back muscles, while your shoulder blades move down your back to support the lifting of your sternum. Your arms form your upper foundation by pressing firmly into the ground.

In other words, backbends can be better understood as the backward bending of the entire body. Yet your spine remains the central focus, as it is the epicenter for emotions, feelings, and energy. The esoteric anatomy of the body locates the chakras, or energy centers, at certain key points along the spine. Go to any chiropractor, and you will see the importance he or she places on keeping the spinal column healthy. Any obstruction in the vertebrae can yield disastrous and paralyzing effects on your life. Yoga asks you to have consciousness within every vertebra. Backbends teach you to lift, extend, create space, and bend deeply by using that space between the joints.

As you work deeply with your spinal column, you may begin to confront all types of issues. There is the pain of asking an area of your lower or upper back that may be used to rounding forward to extend backward. If you spend a good amount of time hunched over your desk, then learning to move your spine in an arched, extended pattern will challenge your entire notion of physicality. If you do it over an extended period, it will not only free up new patterns of movement but also protect the health of your spine throughout your life with safe and proven methods. Despite the healing benefits of backbends, it is this very process of opening and bending that stirs the emotional pot. Many people experience intense muscular pain when working with backbends and even in a simple Urdhva Mukha Svanasana. Muscular pain is relatively safe to work with under the supervision of a teacher who can check your alignment in the pose. It often occurs along the long erector spinae in the back.

These are postural muscles that work to set your daily pose, among other things. People who perpetually experience pain in backbends must look at postural alignment both in their yoga practice and in their daily lives. When you ask your body to move in an unfamiliar way, pain is usually associated with it. Just as when you ask yourself to break your routine and move way outside the box, there is often an ample amount of mental anguish. By contrast, sharp, pinching pain in the vertebrae is a very different type of pain, and you should not try to work with it. Address it and have it diagnosed immediately. If you feel a sharp, pointy pain in your spine during any pose, back off from the movement.

Your hips determine the base point of your spine's ability to move backward. The iliopsoas and hip flexors are two of the major muscle groups whose flexibility is crucial here. If these muscles are tight, then the degree to which you will be able to tilt your pelvis and open your hip joints will decrease. Sometimes lower back stiffness and pain stem from tightness in the iliopsoas and hip flexors. Moving your tailbone forward is important in preventing your lumbar vertebrae from being compressed while moving backward. But it is a movement that is often misunderstood. If you have an injury in your lower back, tuck your tailbone under strongly to protect and avoid the affected area during practice. However, tucking the tailbone also encourages a flattening of the lumbar region, which is not good for deep backbends. For these poses, the tailbone should move forward to direct the weight of your pelvis over the solid foundation of your legs. Then the iliac crests tilt forward to encourage a slightly forward tilt in your pelvis. This action is controlled by the pelvic floor and the strength of your legs. The movement does not flip your tailbone out but activates a rocking of the sacrum that gives space to your lower back and pelvis. This movement is called sacral nutation and indicates that the top of the sacrum tilts forward and into the pelvis, thereby allowing you to use the sacroiliac joints in a similar manner to a spinal process. The ability to open the front of your hips and pelvis is often connected with the ability to move forward in life with a powerful thrust. By allowing your musculature to relax, release, and lengthen, you gain the greater range of motion necessary to literally send your hips forward while you bend your back.

Your shoulders form the upper support for your spine in backbends. Being much more mobile than your hip joints, your shoulder girdle can move in ways that are more likely to facilitate poses and are also more likely to create pain. Working with a knowledgeable teacher who has a keen understanding of alignment will help you dramatically with safe shoulder alignment when you progress to deep backbends. Understood as the gateway to the heart, the shoulders can protect, stabilize, release, reach, extend, get stuck, collapse, give out, and break down. Sometimes tight shoulders prevent you from experiencing the joy of spinal mobility, even if your vertebrae are flexible and strong. When you lift into a backbend, keep your shoulders rolled down your back and rotated externally. Align your wrists, elbows, and shoulders over each other, and avoid turning your hands inward or bending your elbows out to the side. Squeeze your elbows toward each other while pressing firmly into the floor through your fingertips and hands.

During the process of opening your spine, hips, and shoulders in backbends, some common and intense negative emotions such as fear, anxiety, sadness, claustrophobia, suffocation, and anger crop up. Some equally common and intense positive sensations such as joy, happiness, trust, release, surrender, peace, heightened energy, and true power can also emerge. The process of accepting your experience of pain in poses like backbends is often simply about learning not to run away from the physical pain and emotional upheaval. When you feel these emotions, remember that they are temporary and focus on breathing more deeply and relaxing. If you are confronted with an overwhelming emotion or intense physical pain, the best thing to do is focus on your breath. This will give you a pause between the pain stimulus and your automatic desire to run away. From that space of increased awareness you will see more clearly what the appropriate action should be. For example, you will be able to determine whether the pain is muscular or in the joint and whether the emotion is anger or anxiety. Expanding your consciousness one breath at a time is a powerful way to use patience, awareness, and acceptance to move deeper into asanas.

The yoga path is one of freedom, and it is a freedom built on a deep and fundamental acceptance of the truth of life. Life contains suffering, and when you come face-to-face with it, your only logical choice is to accept it, surrender to it, and allow it to teach you one breath at a time.

URDHVA DANURASANA

Lifted Bow Pose

Drishti: Nasagrai (Nose)

This pose (see fig. 8.1) is repeated three times at the end of the Primary Series. Beginners may find it useful to start off with a simple bridge pose instead of attempting a full backbend right away. To try this easy preparatory exercise, inhale and jump through to a seated position following

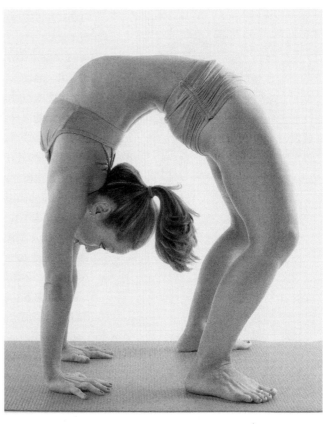

Figure 8.1

the last vinyasa after Setu Bhandasana. Exhale as you lie flat on your back. Bend your knees, placing your feet parallel to the outside of your hips. Hold on to your ankles (see fig. 8.2) or interlace your fingers with your arms straight out on the ground under your pelvis. As you inhale, thrust your heels firmly into the ground, send your knees forward over your ankles, and engage your quadriceps to support the movement. Send your pelvis forward, while pulling in your abdomen and engaging your pelvic floor. Let your sacrum tip into your pelvis, and begin lifting your spine out of your pelvis while elongating your back muscles. Fold your shoulders under your upper chest, raise your sternum, and lift your rib cage forward to potentially make contact with your chin. Take five breaths, paying careful attention to the space you create between your vertebrae while elongating and strengthening your back muscles. Exhale to return all the way to the floor.

If you are using this as an introductory movement, do not force your spine to bend too deeply; just focus on your breath and the feeling of elongation. You can repeat this pose up to three times. If this presents a challenge, stop here and do not proceed with any full backbends.

When you are able, move into the traditional Urdhva Danurasana sequence. Advanced practitioners can skip the simple bridge pose and move directly here from the last vinyasa after Setu Bhandasana. The next three full backbends are done in succession from the floor. You will only come down onto your head for a short break in between. From a prone

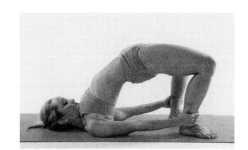

Figure 8.2

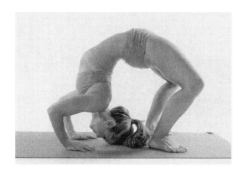

Figure 8.3

position, bend your knees and place your feet parallel to the outside edges of your hips. Place your hands directly under your shoulders, fingers pointing toward your feet, elbows stacked over your palms, and fingers spread wide apart.

On an inhalation, apply the same technique as you did to lift into simple Bridge Pose. Send your knees forward over your ankles, thrust your heels firmly into the ground, and engage your quadriceps to send your pelvis forward over your feet. Tip your sacrum into the pelvis while lifting your spine out of your pelvis. This time, when your body begins to lift off the ground, allow your chest to rise over your hands and roll your shoulder blades down your back to lift your sternum and rib cage. Bending your upper back is crucial to relieving pressure on your lower back, so be sure to distribute the bend equally throughout all your vertebrae and the entire spinal column. After five breaths, come down onto your head as you exhale (see fig. 8.3). Walk your hands slightly closer to your feet, then lift up again as you inhale. Be careful not to lift your heels, or you will lose your connection to the ground. A healthy sign of good backbend technique is to feel an intense burning sensation in your quadriceps but no pinching in your spine or lower back. Think about the inhalation creating space in your joints and the exhalation using the space to go deeper. Be careful not to push too hard and hurry the motion. Give your spine the time it needs to open, and be gentle with yourself. At the same time, find your limit of flexibility and strength, and work to go deeper in a healthy way.

Exhale and come down onto your head, walking your hands in toward your feet again. Inhale and lift up for the last repetition. Hold each backbend for at least five breaths. Since breathing is sometimes shortened during backbends, you could increase the number of breaths to eight or increase the repetitions by one or two. If you feel challenged, stop here. Exhale and lower down, inhale and roll over backward into Chakrasana, then jump through to Paschimattanasana.

STANDING UP AND DROPPING BACK

The second portion of the backbend sequence is very hard to perform. Attempt it only when you can easily straighten your arms fully in Urdhva Danurasana and walk your hands slightly in toward your feet. When you shift your weight forward onto your legs, you create the space to walk your hands closer to your feet and learn to stand up.

If you are ready to try, begin in full backbend and walk your hands as far as you can in toward your feet. Be very conscious about keeping the heels firmly planted on the ground. If the heels lift, do not attempt to walk in any farther. Shift your weight forward onto your feet as you inhale, then backward onto your hands as you exhale. Do this at least five times to test the limits of your flexibility and strength. See if you can come all the way onto your fingertips with the heels planted on the ground as you inhale and send weight forward over your feet. If you can do this easily, then you are ready to try Standing Up and Dropping Back. If not, simply try that gentle rocking motion every day to build up your strength and flexibility. If you are working on the rocking motion, think of it less as building momentum and more as a subtle weight transfer forward into the solid foundation of the pelvis, legs, and feet.

Starting in full backbend, walk your hands as close to your feet as possible. Maintain the same principles of healthy alignment as you did in Urdhva Danurasana. Try not to turn your feet outward, but if it is unavoidable, then strongly rotate your thighs inward to help release your sacrum and press strongly into the ball of the big toe. Keep your knees moving forward over your ankles and then begin to transfer your weight forward onto your feet, pressing down into your heels and the base of each big toe. Send your pelvis farther forward, allowing the iliac crests to tilt and reach forward as well. Bring your weight far enough into your legs that you come up onto your fingertips or your hands come off the ground (see fig. 8.7). If you are strong enough, you can transfer your weight forward by pressing into your feet and pulling yourself up with the power of your legs and pelvis. If you are not that strong, you can rock forward and backward to generate just enough momentum to carry you up. Either way, once your hands are floating in the air, there will be a huge temptation to bring your head up. Avoid this at all costs; your head is always the last thing to come up. Instead, let your head and hands hang back, and send your hips forward again until the weight of your torso is stacked over your hips and

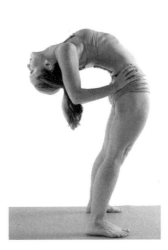
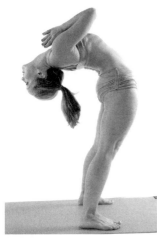
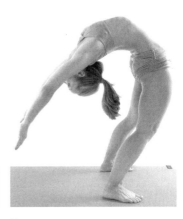
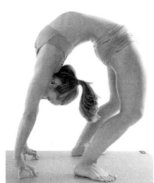

Figure 8.4   *Figure 8.5*   *Figure 8.6*   *Figure 8.7*

feet. Once your chest moves forward over your hips, bring your hands into prayer position in front of your upper chest and your head into alignment over your feet. Try not to splay your feet outward, lift your heels, or widen your stance too much.

When you have risen to standing, it is time try dropping back into Urdhva Danurasana. Some students may find dropping back dramatically easier than standing up. Feel free to try dropping back first if you think that will be easier. Begin with your feet as close to parallel as possible, hip-width or slightly wider apart. Engage your quadriceps while thrusting your weight firmly into the base of each big toe, keeping your legs straight. Place both of your thumbs on your sacrum and push your pelvis forward to take more weight into your big toes (see fig. 8.4). Engage your pelvic floor, draw your abdomen in, and begin lifting your spine out of your pelvis. Allow your sacrum to nutate while lifting and extending your vertebrae. Lift your rib cage to create space as you inhale, and be careful not to let go of that space as you exhale. Lift your sternum as high as possible toward the ceiling. Roll your shoulders down your back. If you feel challenged, stay in this position for five breaths and then inhale to return to standing. If you feel confident here, then continue.

Place your hands in prayer position at the level of your sternum and drop your head back, breathing freely and fully (see fig. 8.5). Be careful to keep the elongation in your spine, as you no longer have the support of your hands at your sacrum to keep your hips moving forward and remind your lower back to lengthen. If this is challenging, stay here for five breaths, then inhale and return to standing. If you feel confident here and have no painful sensations in your back, then continue.

Raise your hands over your head while drawing your shoulder blades down your back (see fig. 8.6). Keep your head dropped back while pushing your pelvis farther forward and thrusting more weight into your feet. Allow a slight bend in your knees, but keep your heels firmly grounded. Look for your mat and hold this position for five breaths. Do not be surprised if you feel as though you cannot breathe; nevertheless, try to breathe fully into your rib cage and allow your lungs to expand. If you can comfortably hold this position for five breaths, see your mat, and think clearly, then you are ready to drop all the way back to the floor. If you feel dizzy, be sure to gaze at one point. If you feel nauseated, breathe deeper and continue.

Find a spot on your mat on which to focus. Exhale as you prepare your arms for landing by spreading your fingers and very slightly bending the elbows, and allow your hands to drop to the floor. Do *not* rush this process. Be happy if it takes a few years or a few lifetimes to master this movement. When you do decide to try it, remember to keep your weight moving forward into your feet, your spine supported by the lift through your core muscles, and your chest lifted to elongate your upper back. When you drop your hands to the floor, it is crucial that you do not literally *drop* them; if you do, you will take too much pressure in your wrists and risk hitting your head. Think of it more like placing your hands on the floor while your legs support the weight of your body.

After you have successfully dropped back, inhale and stand up again. Repeat this up-and-down motion three times. With practice, you will refine the movement until it is fluid, graceful, and easy. Eventually, you will perform it in three linked continuously flowing breaths: exhale down — inhale up — exhale down — inhale up — exhale down — inhale up. However, that is a very advanced movement, and you should not try it before you are ready. If you are practicing with a teacher, wait for assistance before going deeper.

Coming out of the pose from a standing position, if you are practicing at home, you can skip the vinyasa that indicates you should roll over backward, and simply sit down and perform Paschimattanasana. Or you can lie down as you exhale, inhale and roll backward through Chakrasana, and continue the vinyasa.

Paschimattanasana

Seated Forward Bend

Drishti: Padhayoragrai (Toes)

Either jump through to a seated position on an inhalation or sit down from standing backbends. Apply the same forward bend techniques as you did in Chapter 7. The intention of this pose differs slightly as it is meant as a counterstretch to the backbend. In Ashtanga Yoga, we consider it mandatory to release all the back muscles after deep backbends in order to keep the spine healthy. Do not rush the forward bend. Keep your abdomen and pelvic floor engaged, keep the inner integrity of pose intact, and ignore the temptation to just collapse forward. Think consciously about releasing your back muscles into the supportive framework along the front of your body. Lengthen your spine on an inhalation and use the exhalation to help make your transition into the finishing poses smoother (see fig. 8.8).

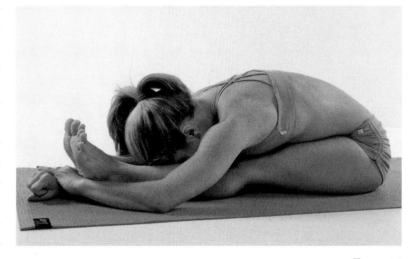

Figure 8.8

This is often the time when the emotions stirred during deep backbends will rise to the surface. If you feel the need to cry during this forward bend, allow your emotions to flow without indulging them. Remain calm and just observe what you feel in a nonjudgmental manner. Stay in the bend for ten breaths, then inhale and straighten your spine. Exhale and settle into the movement. Inhale and lift up; exhale and jump back.

9

Finishing Poses: Entering the Inner Space

TRANSITIONING FROM THE HEIGHTENED FLEXIBILITY, strength, and cardiovascular challenges of the Primary Series and backbend sequence creates a natural shift from hard work to healing space. The finishing poses should be done with minimal force and an attitude of relaxation and ease.

Meant to seal the energy of the practice into your body and mind, the finishing poses restore balance on multiple levels. Since asanas work with the energetic pathways of the body, it is crucial to breathe deeply and take your time throughout the entire finishing pose sequence. It is not just a cool-down routine to be skipped if you do not have time. Always leave enough time in every yoga session to perform the finishing poses and the final relaxation. Although it is best to go through the entire sequence of poses in each session, if you are brand-new to the practice, you may perform only the last three poses of the finishing sequence and the final relaxation until you progress deeper into the Ashtanga Yoga method. If you are performing half of the Primary Series, you are certainly ready for a full finishing pose sequence.

Practically speaking, the finishing poses are meant to be performed by everyone, every day, with two notable exceptions. Pregnant women are advised to modify the inverted postures based on their own unique experience at different times during their pregnancy. Menstruating women should not perform inverted poses of long duration, since the flow of energy in the body is downward during that time. Inversions can disturb the natural flow of the body during this time. Additionally, the psoas muscle sits directly adjacent to the ovaries, and inverted poses demand a deep application of the bandhas, so this is contraindicated during menses. In fact, women should rest for the first three or the heaviest days of their menstrual cycle. When they return to practice, they can perform all noninverted poses normally.

Having dedicated time at the end of your daily practice gives you a chance to check the state of your body and mind after you complete the rigorous yoga routine. Simply taking time to allow yourself to feel the effects of the practice on your emotional, physical, and spiritual state provides you with an honest mirror to the inner body. This careful turning inward of the mind toward the subtlety within is the deepest goal of yoga. The finishing poses are the perfect chance to allow your mind to become more meditative in focus and intention. One easy way to ensure that you are focusing inward is to be conscious of the expression on your face. If you notice yourself furrowing your brow or squinting with effort, soften your expression and look for more subtlety within.

Begin this portion of the series by lying flat on your back for five deep breaths while keeping your body still, your legs and arms outstretched, and your eyes only slightly open. Before starting the finishing poses, allow a neutral, five-breath transition from the work of the Ashtanga Yoga Primary Series. Lying in this neutral, easy position also gives you a chance to stabilize your breath and regain conscious control of the length and quality of each inhalation and exhalation, extending and deepening them. This will help you calm your mind and body and turn your attention even deeper within.

Whereas the cleansing and purifying work of the Primary Series aims to develop intense internal fire, the finishing poses transform the fire of purification into the spiritual fire of awakening. Keeping your mind centered and calm throughout this sequence is essential for success. Additionally, if you work deeply with the poses of any Ashtanga series, the finishing poses will ensure your body's health and prevent injury. The finishing poses are done one after another with a jump back and a jump through between each sequence. This differs from the seated poses, which have a jump back and a jump through between each pose within each sequence. Stringing the poses together allows more of their energy to accumulate, while excluding the vinyasas between each movement helps the body cool down. When done correctly and with the right attitude of relaxation, the finishing poses produce a deeply healing effect that calms the nervous system, protects the joints, and encourages a healthy and spiritually open mind.

These poses are generally easier and less challenging than those of the Primary Series. They are some of the most essential poses of the entire yoga tradition, and their benefits cannot be overstated. They provide some of the deepest healing available, and you will only receive these benefits if you commit yourself fully to practicing these poses every day of your practice.

Such daily practice creates an inner stillness of mind and spirit. Cultivating a meditative awareness of the inner body throughout this sequence is essential to reaping the long-term benefits of practice. This series of poses creates an end point to the practice just as Surya Namaskara creates a starting point. These poses, along with the standing poses, are performed regardless of which series or group of poses you are working on. The main focus of the finishing poses is on inversions and the healing effect of such asanas. My teacher, Sri K. Pattabhi Jois, would often talk about a substance that he described as the "nectar of life" (*amritabindhu*). He said that the Upanishads (sacred spiritual texts) indicated that one drop of this substance is made after about a month of yoga practice if you eat good-quality food. After six months of practice, one small drop of the highest form of this purified energy of life will be stored in the center of your head, at the energy center known as *sahasrara chakra* (crown chakra). Jois would say that this is the minimum amount of time that a new student needs to practice in order to experience life changes. When you can hold inversions easily for a long time, in comfort, and with deep breathing, the pace at which the vital life essence is created is accelerated, and the pace at which it is destroyed is decreased. In daily life, we often spend this spiritual essence on simple daily tasks and lose the luster of our spirit in the world.

The finishing poses are the best place to feel the accumulation of new spiritual energy. When you hold your body upside down for long periods of time, the amritabindhu collects in the part of your brain that is associated with spiritual growth and awakening. Here, gravity works in reverse, so the downward pressure on your organs is reduced. While the amritabindhu is one of yoga's many esoteric concepts of spiritual awakening, others may notice an inner glow in advanced practitioners. Their physical body houses their spirit with grace and the light of knowledge shines out. Without careful cultivation of the vital life essence, this inner glow is more a dream than a reality. But with daily practice, even things that at first seem strange can become real-world experiences. Regular practice of the finishing poses bridges the gap between the physical and the spiritual and gives you the opportunity to experience your spiritual energy every day.

SALAMBA SARVANGASANA

Shoulderstand

Drishti: Nasagrai (Nose)

Start off lying on the floor with a straight spine. Prepare your core muscles to lift your body weight off the ground with a careful application of the bandhas (see Chapter 10 for an explanation of bandhas). Lift directly into the pose on an inhalation. Thrust your upper arms into the ground and

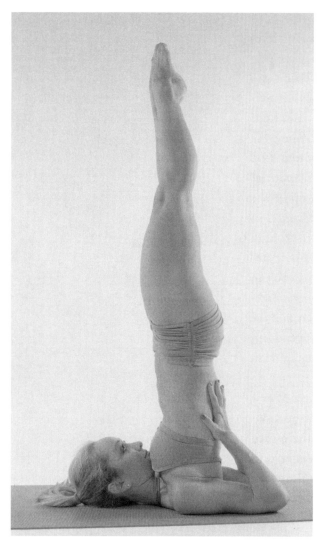

Figure 9.1

engage the bandhas as you send the weight of your lower body over the foundation of your upper arms. As you lift your hips off the ground, send them over your torso and immediately roll your shoulders under your body. Be careful not to squeeze your shoulder blades together, as this may cause unnecessary tension in your neck. Simply allow your shoulders and upper arms to press into the ground and under your now lifted body. Place your hands at the middle of your back to help support your spine. You may find it useful to roll slightly from side to side to let your arms rotate fully underneath your body. Once you have completed the lift, your feet, legs, hips, rib cage, and shoulders should all be in a straight line and your body should be perpendicular to the ground (see fig. 9.1).

Bring your elbows closer together until they are in line with your shoulders; any closer than that is not necessary. When your elbows are farther apart than your shoulders, it is a good indication that your shoulders may be tight and need some additional stretching. Shoulderstand is a safe place for you to gain this flexibility. Make sure that you actively press your fingers and hands into your lower back to provide stability and the right amount of activation. Do *not* press your neck into the ground. Instead, thrust down with your shoulders and upper arms, making the pose a true "shoulder" stand. Keep your neck in line with your spine while gazing at your nose. By pressing your chin against the sternoclavicular joint you perform *jalandhara bandha* (chin lock), which helps regulate the flow of energy in this pose.

If you find it impossible to lift directly into the pose, or if this lift stresses your neck, there is another easy but nontraditional way to enter Shoulderstand. Start by lying flat on your back. Instead of lifting straight up to the full pose, press your hands into the floor, fold your body at the hip joints, and roll your legs over your head. Rest the tips of your toes on the ground to provide support, and then roll your body from side to side to deepen the rotation in your shoulders. Line up your elbows with your shoulder blades, place your hands on your midback for support, and lift one leg at a time. If you still feel pain in your neck, try placing a blanket under your arms and letting your neck hang over the edge toward the floor. Whichever version you perform, do your best to keep the curve of your neck off the ground so you do not damage the cervical vertebrae.

To support the weight of your body, engage your pelvic floor and activate the bandhas. Lift your hips higher with each breath, using the strength of your whole body to raise yourself strongly off the ground. Draw your ribs in so that your torso lifts itself as well. Point your toes firmly and reach for the ceiling with your feet. Actively press the bases of your big toes together so your thighs rotate inward slightly. Engage the inside of your quadriceps to encourage this rotation. Try to feel that the entire length of both legs is linked energetically as one long, clean line as well as being connected to your pelvic floor and torso.

Sarvangasana stretches your upper back and neck while strengthening the bandhas and your core muscles. It is also the most easily accessible inverted pose. Stretching your upper back demands that you release any tension around your trapezius muscles, an area where many people hold chronic stress. To move the joints of your upper back and neck freely, it is necessary to release the state of mind associated with long-term stress. Your nervous system must relax. The process of lifting your own weight completely off the ground for prolonged periods of time builds inner confidence and self-esteem, and it ultimately cures fear-based stress responses. To lift your own body weight off the ground, you need to cultivate a deep inner strength. Regular practice of Sarvangasana builds the foundational elements needed to be both physically and mentally strong enough to perform much harder inverted positions. Careful application of safe anatomical techniques can easily be integrated for all practitioners to establish the foundations needed for harder movements. This pose also induces deep purification of the pineal glands and the lymphatic system. Try to hold the pose for at least fifteen to twenty-five breaths. Proceed directly into the next posture.

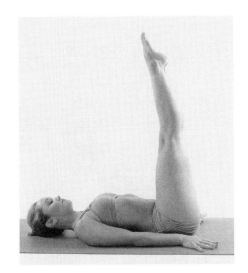

Figure 9.2

One final modification for menstruating women or individuals with serious neck injuries is a pose called Viparita Karani, or Legs-Up-the-Wall Pose (see fig. 9.2). For the easiest version of this pose, lie on the floor with your pelvis as close to a wall as possible. Straighten your legs up the wall and lock the sides of your heels and big toes together. Keep your feet flexed. For a slightly more challenging version without the wall, lie with your back flat on the ground and lift your legs straight up from your pelvis so that they are perpendicular to your torso. Apply all the same techniques already outlined for Sarvangasana. Hold for between ten and twenty breaths. Proceed directly to Matsyasana.

BENEFITS

Regulates glandular functions, including those of the thyroid and parathyroid

Treats asthma, bronchitis, and throat disorders

Soothes the nervous system

Treats depression and anxiety

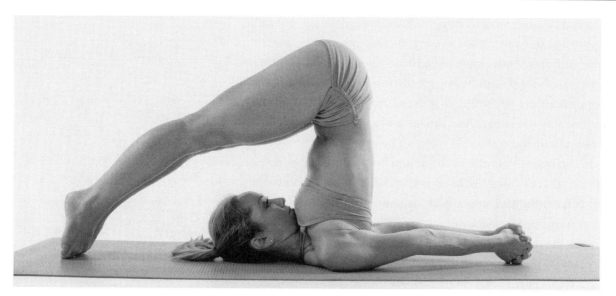

Figure 9.3

Treats urinary tract infections, uterine disorders, and hernias
Aligns the spine
Stretches the neck
Tones the legs and pelvic floor
Improves digestion and circulation

HALASANA

Plow Pose

Drishti: Nasagrai (Nose)

Halasana immediately follows Sarvangasana and continues its deep healing work and subtle focus on the inner body. Halasana is a semi-inverted pose that is deeply relaxing and requires less effort than Sarvangasana. It can be performed easily and comfortably by nearly everyone. Enter this pose directly from the one preceding, creating a cumulative effect of your spiritual work.

Lower your hands to the ground behind your back. Keep your shoulders locked in place beneath your upper body and your cervical spine fully raised off the floor. On an exhalation, slowly change the position of your legs drawing in your abdomen and allowing your hip joints to flex deeply; point your toes, touch the bases of the big toes together, and keep your legs straight. Ideally, the line of your legs from hip to toe is at an angle greater than ninety degrees so that the tops of your feet rest firmly on the ground. To achieve this alignment, rotate your hip joints internally, engaging your quadriceps and softening your hip flexors. Let your toes rest on the floor, but do not press them down. Just allow the natural point of the toes to extend toward the floor with the strength of your legs. (If you press your toes into the ground, you will take your foot out of full point.) Pointing the toes is a crucial alignment connection that helps the energy flow along the subtle pathways in the body, enabling Halasana to provide maximum effect. Finally, interlock your fingers on the floor and straighten your arms so that your body is now supporting itself with the strength of your torso, arms, and core (see fig. 9.3).

Your spine should be straight in this pose. The deep flexion of the hip joints when your legs are totally engaged allows your toes to reach toward the ground. Avoid rounding your back or forcing your legs down to get your feet on the floor. Keep your abdomen drawn deeply into your body. Since you have a good view of your lower belly at this point, you can be even more aware of the deep work with the bandhas that helps the finishing poses achieve their powerful effect. If you are unable to touch your feet to the ground because your body is too tight, try using your hands to support your lower back instead of clasping them on the floor. Gravity will work on your legs and increase the flexion in your hips if you let your legs dangle in the air. Try to keep your knees totally straight in both versions of the pose, as this increases the flow of energy throughout them and connects them deeply to the interior space of your pelvis.

This pose is a mini-inversion that requires you to lift your spine from within and let each body part be responsible for lifting itself. Be careful not to press your upper neck into the ground; keep your weight supported on your shoulders and upper arms.

This simple pose integrates the work of the Ashtanga Yoga Primary Series by helping bring energy up your spine and stimulating the amritabindhu. Holding the position for a long time helps settle the mind and calm the breath. Place careful emphasis on controlling the length of your inhalations and exhalations so they are equal. Hold this pose for eight breaths. Come down directly into Karnapidasana.

Benefits

Regulates glandular functions, including those of the thyroid
   and parathyroid
Treats asthma, bronchitis, and throat disorders
Soothes the nervous system
Treats depression and anxiety
Treats urinary tract infections, uterine disorders, and hernias
Aligns the spine
Stretches the neck and hamstrings
Tones the legs and pelvic floor
Improves digestion and circulation

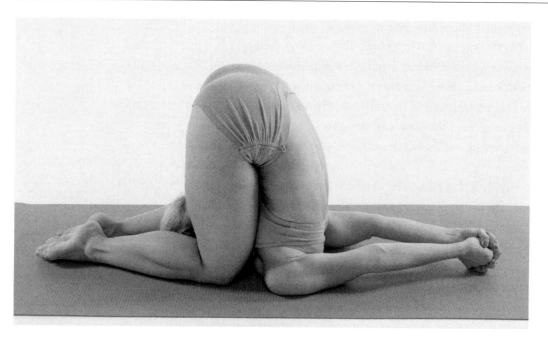

Figure 9.4

KARNAPIDASANA

Ear Pressure Pose

Drishti: Nasagrai (Nose)

Continue the flow created from the beginning of the sequence by entering Karnapidasana directly from Halasana. Bend your knees so that they reach toward the floor and press your knees against your ears; keep your fingers interlocked and your arms outstretched on the floor as they were in Halasana.

Whereas the previous two poses required as straight a spine as possible, this pose involves flexing your spine. To do this safely, you must draw your abdomen in and activate your pelvic floor for the full application of the bandhas (see Chapter 10). The only healthy way to round your back is to give it full support with the muscles on the front side of your body. If you attempt to keep your spine straight in this pose, you will miss the chance to develop your inner strength and increase your awareness of the bandhas. Similarly, if you merely round your back without the support of your front muscles, you will miss the essence of the pose. Use the bandhas to actively lift your spine over your head as explained for Baddha Konasana B in Chapter 7. The torso lifts itself away from the ground, creates space and relieves pressure around the back of the neck, and supports the vertebrae as you go into a deep forward bend. Throughout this pose, the back of your neck should never be flat on the ground. If you feel undue pressure there, use the bandhas to lift your body away from your neck while pressing your shoulders more firmly into the ground, thereby creating space for your cervical vertebrae.

If possible, touch your knees to your ears and the floor at the same time (see fig. 9.4). If you cannot do this, then simply press your knees to your ears as tightly as possible while curving your back inward. Squeezing the ears is crucial for Karnapidasana, because it is meant to heal all imbalances in the ear and inner ear. With the application of equal pressure directly on both ears, the balance centers inside the ears are normalized. If your knees are on the ground, you can also press them down slightly, but the pressure on your ears should remain constant.

If you cannot immediately touch your knees to your ears, draw your stomach in even farther and allow your back to round a little more to increase the flexion of your spine. Do not squeeze your abdomen to get into the pose. If your knees still do not reach, you may find it useful to support your lower back with your hands. If your knees do not touch either your ears or the floor, you might also try draping your arms around the backs of your knees to help bring them into position. Apply this modification only on a temporary basis when it is absolutely necessary, as the pose is more effective when you use only your core strength. If you are able to press your knees into your ears, but your knees still float above the ground, keep your arms outstretched and your fingers interlocked. One helpful modification is to lean your pelvis to one side, placing one knee on the ground for a few breaths and then switch sides. Squeeze your ears with your knees once more, while flexing your spine in a final attempt to bring your knees all the way to the floor.

The weight of your body should be distributed between your hands, shoulders, and the center of the back of your head. You ideally feel an equal distribution of weight between these areas. Most students initially feel challenged to let their weight bear down on their shoulders and the back of their head; however, this is essential for balance in Karnapidasana. Having full control of your weight distribution helps increase your awareness of your body in space and helps relieve the fear associated with being out of balance. Be sure to keep your body supported with core strength and with careful use of the bandhas. Listen to your body and feel the inner energy channels to support the pose.

A further aspect of turning inward evident in this pose is the direction of the sense organs to the inner body. By cutting out sound from the external world, you are invited (and better able) to tune in to the quieter inner channels. See if you can hear your heartbeat, pulse, circulation, or any other sounds in your subtle body. As your powers of concentration become more refined, you will hear and feel more sounds and experiences.

Hold this pose for eight breaths. Come out of it and move directly into the next one, Urdhva Padmasana.

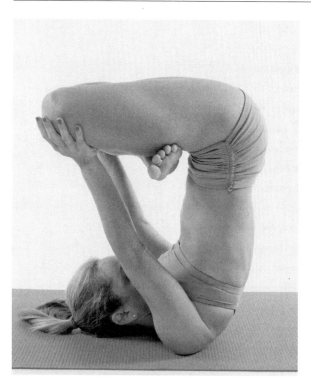

Figure 9.5

BENEFITS

Heals ear disorders such as ringing in ears
Alleviates insomnia and fatigue
Stretches the back muscles
Evens out imbalances and twists, like scoliosis
Tones the pelvic floor

URDHVA PADMASANA

Flying Lotus Pose

Drishti: Nasagrai (Nose)

This pose asks you to perform a full lotus position while balancing upside down. Before you even attempt this, it is a good idea to test your ability to get into lotus position safely and easily while seated. If you find Padmasana difficult to perform while resting in a comfortable seated position, it will be even harder in an inverted pose. Wait until you can do that easier version before you work on the full version of this pose. If lotus position is unattainable now, do not force it. You may do a half-lotus position or simply cross your legs in the air. Decide which modification you will use before you try the pose.

Once you have decided on either full lotus, half-lotus, or no lotus, start from Karnapidasana, lift your legs, and come back into full Sarvangasana. If you need to, use your hands to support your midback. Once you are in Sarvangasana, find your balance and begin entering your chosen cross-legged position. Be sure not to turn or twist your neck while attempting the next series of movements. If your hips are open enough, you may be able to enter lotus position without using your hands. However, most people need a little help to direct their legs and feet to the appropriate places. Entering lotus position from an inverted pose requires that the front of your pelvis be a little more open than it is in the seated version. Be careful and gentle with your body, as there is a lot to oversee throughout this motion. Just as in the seated pose, do not squeeze your knees to get into position and follow the same safety guidelines for getting into lotus.

Start your attempt for full lotus by bringing your left leg toward the back of your body, away from your face to open the hip joint and hip crease. Aim your right foot toward the left hip crease, using an external rotation of the right hip joint to get the foot in place. If necessary, use your hands to guide your right foot down toward the left hip crease. Once your right foot is in place, move your right knee up toward the ceiling, pulling it back and away from your face. Angle your left foot toward the back of your right knee, externally rotating the left hip joint to get it into place. If possible, slide your left foot around your right knee and down toward the right hip crease. If your left foot gets stuck, you can either try to wiggle it and inch the toes around or use your hands. The latter challenges your balance but makes for an easier transition into lotus. If you are working with half-lotus, leave your left foot dangling in the air behind your right knee. If you are working with no lotus, simply cross your ankles in the air.

Once your legs are comfortably folded into place, transfer your weight to your upper shoulders and the back of your head, and lift your hands to your knees. Your balance point in this pose will usually be a little more toward the back of the head and the shoulders than at first seems comfortable. Play around with the balance until you can safely lift your hands off the ground. One way to try is to place one hand firmly on the appropriate knee for five breaths, lower it, and then take another five breaths with the other hand in position. Once you build confidence in your body's ability to balance upside down, you can lift both hands.

Once you can balance safely with both hands touching both knees, straighten your arms and actively press your hands into your knees to lift your lotus position into the air (see fig. 9.5). Ideally, your spine should hold the same position in Urdhva Padmasana that it does in seated Padmasana — as straight as possible with no flexion. If you can easily hold your knees in lotus or half-lotus position, then draw your shoulder blades down your back, strengthen your back muscles to support your body, suck in your abdomen, and stabilize your arms. Regardless of which type of leg position you have chosen, the essential nature of the pose remains intact. Lift yourself as though fully inverted in shoulderstand while keeping your spine as straight as possible. Let your knees rest in the palms of your hands, but avoid putting your full weight into your hands. Let the contact be just enough to establish an energetic connection but not so much so that the work of lifting your spine and body from within is compromised. If you merely let your weight fall into your hands, your neck could receive too much pressure. If you start to feel compression in your neck, lift your body away from the ground with the full strength of each individual part to relieve some of the pressure. In this pose, the spine lengthens in a neutral position, neither extended nor flexed, following the natural curvature of the back.

This pose should feel active and dynamic as well as restful and healing. Once your shoulders and the back of your head are pressed fully into ground, your hands are touching your knees, and the bandhas are lifting you from within, you will be able to find perfect balance. Holding Urdhva Padmasana also helps the subtle energy channels in the center of your brain to open, stimulating the production of the amritabindhu.

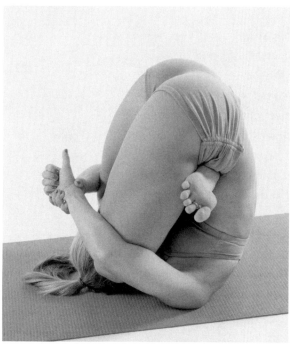

Figure 9.6

Hold this pose for eight breaths. Come directly out of it and into the next one, Pindasana.

BENEFITS

Strengthens bandhas
Increases blood flow to the brain
Strengthens the shoulders
Directs the vital life energy into the central column of the
    sushumna nadi
Calms the nervous system

PINDASANA

Embryo Pose

Drishti: Nasagrai (Nose)

Enter this pose directly from the previous one. Fold your lotus or modified lotus position in toward your body. Lift your spine toward your head, creating space to round your back inward. Imagine that you are curling in on yourself and folding deeply within your inner body to form cavernous openings like the inside of a shell. The physical inward turning stimulates a similar inward turning of the mind. As you begin to feel the inner spaces within your pelvis open, your mind will also open to new levels of spiritual awareness.

From Urdhva Padmasana, try to reach the shins all the way forward until they make contact with the eyebrow. Rather than just resting your legs on your chest or stomach, actively lift your body over your head to create space within your pelvis and abdomen. Use this space to stretch your back muscles while flexing the spine and feeling the inner body. Once you feel balanced, reach your hands around your thighs and hold your wrist or interlace your fingers (see fig. 9.6).

This movement is similar to Baddha Konasana B and demands that you pay attention to the bandhas. It is crucial that throughout this spinal flexion motion your lower belly is drawn in to stabilize your spine and protect your vertebrae. When your abdomen and pelvic floor are engaged, it is easier for your body to lift itself off the ground, and you will develop the strength to jump back, jump through, and perform much more challenging inversions. The intention of this pose is to assist the motion of your spine back toward a dynamic place of strength and ease as well as to deepen the inner work of the finishing poses. You will feel your steady progression to deeper states of consciousness in the inner body. Elongating the breath is a crucial component of the efficacy of this portion of the Ashtanga Yoga series, so pay careful attention to extending and equalizing the length of your inhalations and exhalations.

Hold this pose for eight breaths. Exhale as you unroll and lie down. Move directly into the next pose, Matsyasana.

BENEFITS

Turns the mind inward
Flexes the spine
Strengthens the bandhas
Stimulates the ajna chakra

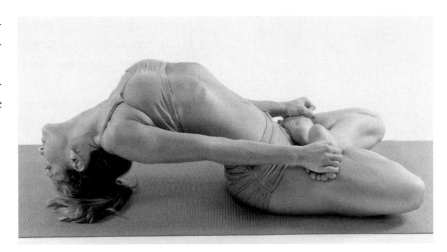

Figure 9.7

MATSYASANA

Fish Pose

Drishti: Broomadhya (Eyebrow center)

Enter this pose directly from the previous one. Place your hands on the ground beside your pelvis, sucking in your abdomen and lifting your body away from the floor. Leaving your head and shoulders on the ground, unroll your spine as though you were unraveling a very delicate ball of string. Control the movement of each vertebra and allow your spine to unfold gently to the ground to assist its full range of motion. Once you are lying prone, place your lotus or modified lotus on the ground so that your knees touch down; do not force them down. Lift and extend your spine as you inhale. You may find it helpful to rest your elbows on the ground as you lift backward to get more height. Finally, place the top of your head on the ground in the same position as when you prepared for Setu Bandhasana and gaze between your eyebrows. You might want to use your hands to reposition your head so that it bends even farther under your neck, increasing the extension of your cervical spine. Remember to engage your neck muscles to lift the vertebrae rather than letting them collapse down.

Moving from the previous two poses into this one will take your spine gently through a full range of motion, from neutral to flexed to extended. Ending with a long extension helps lift the energy in the central column of your body and increase its flow toward the subtle currents that lead to spiritual realization. Be sure to keep your lower abdomen drawn in throughout the movement to both support your spine and allow the energy to rise fluidly along the inner body.

Once you have established a firm foundation in this pose, reach your hands forward and take hold of your feet if they are in lotus position. If you have modified the lotus, place your hands on the tops of your thighs. Straighten your arms while rolling your shoulders down your back to help open and lift your upper chest (see fig. 9.7). Engage your back muscles just as in Urdhva Danurasana and support your spine through its full extension. Press your sit bones into the ground to stabilize your pelvis and consciously apply the bandhas. Tip your sacrum forward into your pelvis while actively lifting your lumbar spine away from the downward thrust of your sit bones. Try to press your knees fully into the floor but do not create tension in your knees. Let the movement of your thighs toward the floor come from opening your hip flexors. Gaze steadily at the space between your eyebrows to help push the energy up your spine.

The main purpose of this pose is to lift energy currents along the subtle body so they can reach the center of spiritual knowingness in the center of your head. Once the vital life force reaches this high level of awareness, a sense of deep peace and integration enters the body and mind. The longer hold required as part of the closing sequence promotes the steady accumulation of energy.

Hold this pose for eight breaths. Come out directly into the next pose, Uttana Padasana.

BENEFITS

Extends and strengthens the spine
Lifts the life energy along the central column of the sushumna nadi
Opens the ajna chakra (psychic center) and throat center
Encourages abdominal support of the spine
Treats fatigue, anxiety, and respiratory dysfunction

UTTANA PADASANA

Extended-Foot Pose

Drishti: Broomadhya (Eyebrow center)

Enter this pose directly from the previous one. Keeping your spine fully extended, release your legs from the lotus or folded position. Extend your legs up and out at a forty-five-degree angle to the floor. Release your arms and reach forward to form a forty-five-degree angle with them as well. Touch your palms together and make sure that your legs and arms are parallel to each other. To counteract the pressure on your lower back, draw your abdomen in strongly, push your sit bones into the ground, engage your lower back muscles to lift your spine out of your pelvis, and engage your legs so they lift with their own strength (see fig. 9.8). Any pressure in your neck is counterbalanced by the forward reach of the legs.

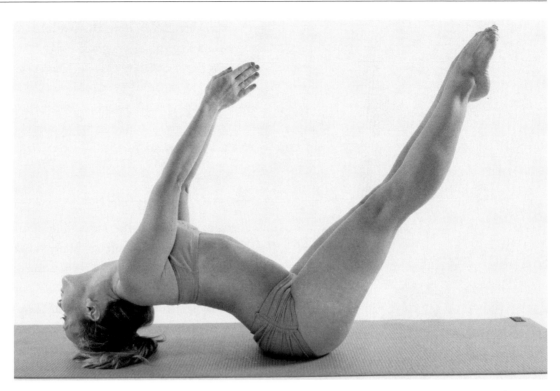

Figure 9.8

This is a challenging pose that demands your full attention physically as well as energetically. It brings the energy even more strongly up your spine and into the central column of your body so that the next inverted pose is easier and your degree of realization is deeper. It also strengthens your back muscles to ease any tension created during deep backbends.

Gaze strongly at the space between your eyebrows. If the tension in your spine and neck is too intense, you may lie flat on the ground and simply lift your arms and legs without the spinal extension. However, try the extension if at all possible, because it is crucial to the benefits of this pose. Hold this pose for eight breaths.

Come out by lowering your back to the floor, while keeping your legs raised as you exhale. You may pause for a moment to let your back flatten and release, but keep your legs in the air. Place your hands under your shoulders, suck in your belly, draw the lower ribs toward the center, and lift your legs over your head as in Halasana, except this time you curl your toes under to flex the feet. On an inhalation, lift your hips over your head and roll over backward, performing Chakrasana. Exhale as you land in Chaturanga Dandasana.

BENEFITS

Stimulates the thyroid
Strengthens the spine, legs, and back

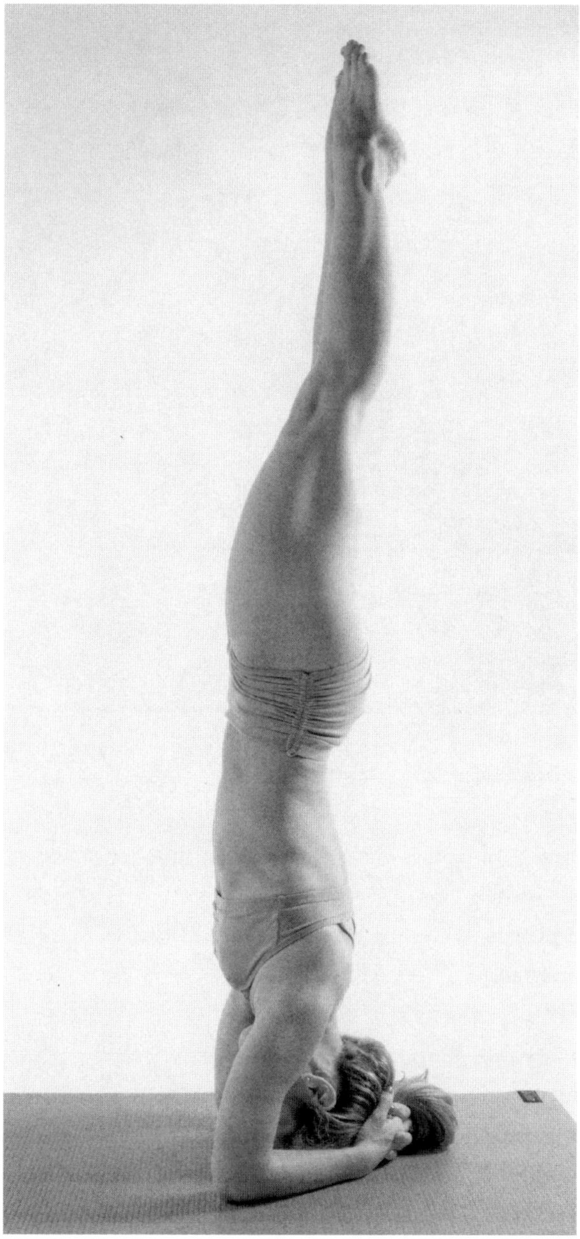

Figure 9.9

Lifts the life energy along the central column of the sushumna nadi

Opens the ajna chakra (psychic center) and throat center

Sirsasana

Headstand

Drishti: Nasagrai (Nose)

Sirsasana is one of the most ubiquitous poses in the Hatha Yoga tradition, and there are many variations. In the finishing sequence of Ashtanga Yoga, we use the easiest and most accessible version (see fig. 9.9). Traditional yoga texts state that you must remain in a headstand for at least three to five minutes before you begin to feel the healing benefit, but be sure to build up to that duration over time. Your spine is ideally in a neutral position when you are in the full pose, and the strength of your shoulder girdle creates a solid foundation for your body. Many people make the mistake of putting too much weight on the head in Sirsasana instead of applying an integrated approach to balance, stability, and strength. Jois always said that headstands were to strengthen the shoulders on a physical level and steady the mind on a spiritual one. The deeper spiritual benefits of this pose come from the balanced attitude you maintain while attempting it and the strength you need to hold it for a long time at the end of your practice. Energy can only enter your body's central column if your mind and body are open and strong. The longer you are able to hold the pose, the stronger the effects will be. By stimulating the glandular and endocrine systems, the headstand is a healing pose that works on many layers of the body.

Start in a kneeling position; place your forearms on the ground. Cup your elbows with your hands to determine the correct distance between the elbows. Maintain this distance but interlock your fingers while keeping your palms open. Your arms should now form a kind of tripod. Engage your deltoids and latissimus dorsi muscles, and draw your shoulder blades down your back and away from each other. Feel this solid foundation in your arms before you move forward, and do not continue if you do not feel stable in your shoulder girdle. If you do, place your head on the floor at the apex of the tripod, in the open space between your palms. Grip your head with your fingers, which are still interlaced, with the pinkies pressed into the ground. Keep your shoulders firm and your arms activated while you thrust down more firmly with your elbows and hands; use the strength in your latissimus dorsi muscles for support. Be sure there is ample space between your ears and your shoulders just as in Adho Mukha Svanasana.

Having established this firm foundation, straighten your legs, pushing up onto your toes (see fig. 9.10). Walk your feet in as close to your head as you can, but be careful not to lift your elbows off the ground. Press even harder into your solid foundation, strengthen your shoulder girdle, and send your hips forward over that foundation. Initiate the movement by feeling the sacrum and the back moving over the shoulders. Inhale as your hips move past your elbows to a point where a natural feeling of liftedness wants to happen in your pelvis. Do not immediately try to lift or kick up; keep moving your pelvis forward until your feet get lighter and lighter and ultimately rise off the ground naturally. If your hamstrings are open, you can continue this movement with straight legs. If your hamstrings are too tight to let you walk close into your head, bend your knees while you walk in. If you are having a hard time lifting off the ground, draw one knee to your chest and squeeze it in while sending your pelvis forward until the other foot naturally wants to lift. If you are able to balance with both knees at your chest (see fig. 9.11), this is a great intermediary step to doing the full pose. If you cannot lift both feet off the ground, then stay in the preparation pose for five or ten breaths. At the end of those five or ten breaths you might gently bend your knees and see if you can rock onto you arms with a small, soft jump that sends your pelvis forward. Do not jump with a lot of force.

If you are able to lift with either straight legs or both knees bent, allow your feet to go up steadily while you breathe calmly. Do not jerk your body or lose your foundation. Keep pressing into your arms and sending your pelvis forward while drawing your abdomen in and engaging your pelvic floor. When you reach the point where your thighs are about parallel to the ground and your feet are floating in the air, begin to bring your hips back over the center of your tripod foundation. Suck your abdomen in and stack your hips over your ribs and torso; your whole body is stacked in the center of your tripod foundation. Keep pressing firmly into your elbows, engaging your deltoids and latissimus dorsi muscles. Pull your abdomen in and strengthen and straighten your legs, reaching your toes up toward the sky. Remain calm and balanced and gaze at the tip of your nose.

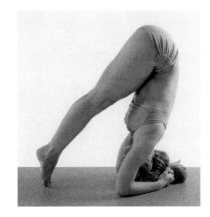

Figure 9.10

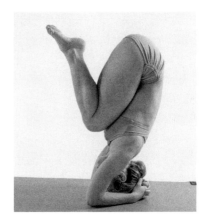

Figure 9.11

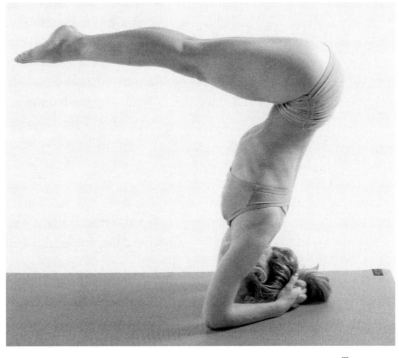

Figure 9.12

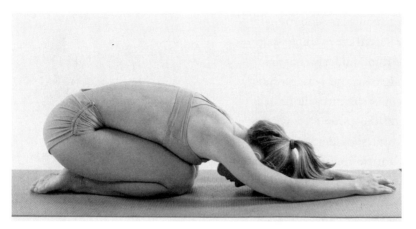

Figure 9.13

Hold this pose for fifteen to twenty-five breaths — around five minutes — or as long as possible. Begin to lower your legs to a half-inverted position so that they are parallel to the ground and your pelvis is pushed back-ward, slightly off-center in the same halfway-up position as when you entered the pose. Keep your legs as straight as possible (see fig. 9.12). Consciously suck your belly and lower ribs in and do the work of the pose from the front side of your body rather than just arching your spine and overworking your back muscles. Let your pelvis be hollow to create the space for a natural pelvic lift. Hold this pose for ten breaths, then lift up to a full headstand again and come to balance.

Once you find your balance, lower yourself all the way down to the ground and enter Balasana, or Child's Pose (see fig. 9.13), in which you bring your knees together, draw your belly in, and rotate your thighs slightly inward. Rest your forehead on the floor, rest your sit bones on your heels, close your eyes, and stretch your arms out above your head. Relax and turn your mind inward. Stay in this pose for five breaths, then jump back to Chaturanga Dandasana as you exhale.

Benefits

Builds strength throughout the body and mind
Calms the nervous system
Draws the life energy up along the central column of the sushumna nadi
Increases blood flow to the brain
Stimulates the pineal and pituitary glands
Improves digestion
Drains the lymph system
Relieves swelling in the legs
Increases self-confidence and inner strength

Baddha Padmasana / Yoga Mudra

Bound Lotus Pose / Sacred Seal

Drishti: Nasagrai (Nose)

Baddha Padmasana and Yoga Mudra are considered to be a sacred seal. The intention of these poses is to complete the ritual of the Ashtanga Yoga practice and turn the full attention of the mind inward. Once this happens, the spiritual body awakens and the vital life force flows freely. The result will be a calm mind, a healed body, and an inner glow.

Enter this pose by jumping through to a sitting position on an inhalation. Exhale as you take your right foot into half-lotus position, and bring your left foot up to full lotus following the instructions on safe external rotation of the hip joint in seated poses (see Chapter 7). Try to let your heels spread away from each other so they align on either side of your navel without touching it. If possible, allow your knees to touch the ground, but do not force them. Once you feel at ease in this pose, reach around your back to hold your left foot with your left hand and your right foot with your right hand. This movement literally binds your lotus and seals the energy lines of the body (see fig. 9.14). You do not need to cross your elbows in back, just reach your arms around enough to clasp your feet firmly. To do this, you must reach from deep within your shoulder joint, just as you did in Supta Kurmasana. This movement ensures that your chest and its corresponding energy centers are open to the free flow of subtle energy.

If you are unable to perform the lotus position, use either half-lotus or a simple cross-legged pose. Take your hands behind your back and hold on to your elbows to simulate the bind. If you are able to get into the lotus position but cannot bind your feet, try wrapping a towel around each foot and holding those rather than just clasping your elbows. If you grip each towel firmly, this activation will help you open your shoulders. If you are able to grab one foot but not the other, try placing a towel around the foot you cannot grab and alternating feet each day. Over time, your shoulders will open. Hold Baddha Padmasana for only one breath to prepare for the next pose.

Having established this bind or modified bind, fold forward on an exhalation to enter Yoga Mudra (see fig. 9.15). Lift your belly inward and hollow out your pelvis. If you can do lotus position easily, you can even press your heels into your belly to assist the hollowing motion. Keep a sense of grounding in your sit bones, although you may allow them to rise slightly off the ground. Reach your spine up and over your feet and aim your chin toward the ground. If you cannot reach your chin to the ground, then touch your forehead to the floor or let it hover in the air while reaching toward the floor. Elongate your spine forward in a slight flexion while the muscles in the front of your body provide support from underneath. This pose firmly cements all the

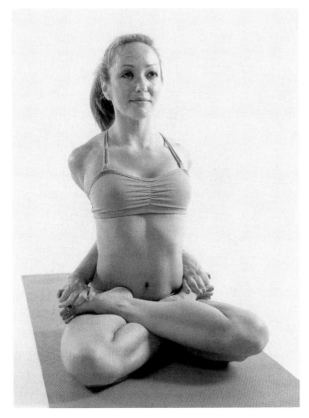

Figure 9.14

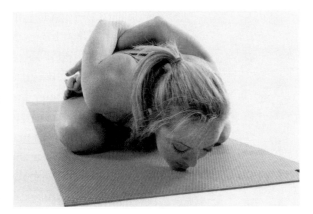

Figure 9.15

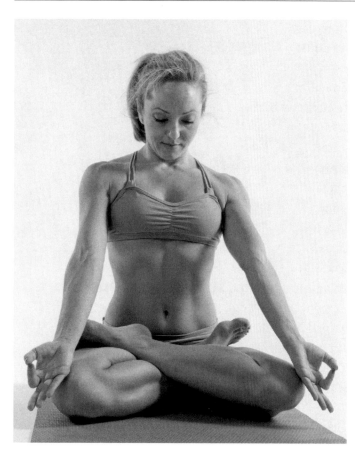

Figure 9.16

learning and energy you have experienced during the practice session into your body and mind. Consciously lengthen your inhalations and exhalations while you are in this pose.

Hold the pose for ten breaths. Come up and go directly into the next pose, Padmasana.

BENEFITS

Opens the hips and shoulders
Directs the mind toward the inner body
Improves digestion
Increases awareness of the bandhas
Treats arthritis

PADMASANA

Full Lotus Pose

Drishti: Nasagrai (Nose)

Full lotus position tests your spiritual energy and intention with the Ashtanga Yoga method. If performed with power and integrity, Padmasana can be the gateway to far deeper states of consciousness than any other pose. It is also used as a preparation for meditation and breathing exercises.

To enter this pose, inhale and sit up from Yoga Mudra, release your hands, and keep your legs in the lotus position. Roll your shoulders down your back, lift your chest and heart center, and straighten your elbows. Turn your palms outward, holding your hands in the gesture known as yoga mudra (which is different than the pose you just held). On each hand, place the tips of your thumb and index finger together to form a link that symbolizes the unity of personal identity with the cosmic, universal life force. Stretch out the three remaining fingers on each hand; they represent mastery over the three gunas (sattva, rajas, tamas), which are manifestations of the forms of nature and are in a state of eternal flux.

While maintaining Padmasana, you must pay careful attention to the inner work of your pelvis. Emphasize the bandhas, and focus your mind deep within the cavernous pelvic regions. At the end of each inhalation and exhalation, bring your mind into true contact with your inner body. See if you can feel the natural application of the pelvic floor contraction as your breath moves in and out of your body. With conscious intention, keep your abdomen drawn in and apply even more pressure to your pelvic floor muscles with each breath. In doing so, you will charge the power center inside your pelvis and fully pump spiritual energy up your spine. Lengthen the inhalation and exhalation even more while drawing in on the bandhas; aim for a full ten-second inhalation and exhalation.

Ground your sit bones firmly into the floor while lifting your spine away from your pelvis. Each inhalation lifts your sternoclavicular joint (at the junction of the sternum and clavicles) toward your chin. Let your chin gently rest downward. On the exhalation, there will be a space between your chin and your chest. Keep your abdomen strongly drawn in throughout the breathing process. Make sure that your spine is in its natural position throughout this pose, neither overly extended nor flexed. Gaze at the tip of your nose (see fig. 9.16). Breathe deeply and strongly, feeling the full power of the Ashtanga Yoga method. Let the sound of your breath be the full expression of your vital life energy, and feel the central channel of your spirit body being charged with this power.

Hold the pose for ten breaths. Proceed immediately to the next pose.

BENEFITS

Opens all the chakras
Stabilizes the pelvis
Increases the subtle flow of energy
Equalizes the breath
Calms the nervous system
Opens the hips and shoulders

UTPLUTIH

Sprung-Up Pose

Drishti: Nasagrai (Nose)

Literally translated as "sprung-up," Utplutih uses the power of the charged inner body to spring upward both physically and energetically. It is a true test of mental and spiritual endurance, and most students find it overwhelming. But with regular practice and good technique, anyone can perform it and receive its benefits. The key to mastering this pose is your willingness to do the inner strength work no matter what it takes. Every student of yoga wants to come down and quit early here, but the deeper lesson is about developing the determination to stay the course regardless of how arduous it seems at first. When you master this pose, you will have tapped into one of the deepest sources of strength available through physical yoga practice.

Place your hands on the floor in front of your pelvis and about mid-thigh. Spread your fingers apart and consciously build a strong foundation

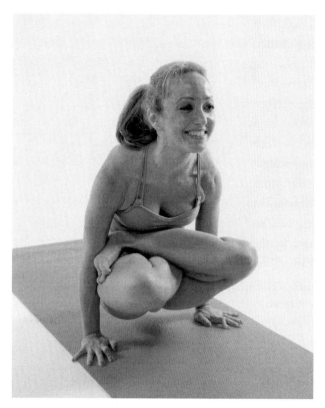

Figure 9.17

with your shoulders. Engage your deltoids, latissimus dorsi muscles, serratus anterior muscles, and rhomboids while you prepare to lift your body off the ground. Flex your hip joints, squeeze the lower ribs toward the center, draw your abdomen in strongly, and engage your pelvic floor to lift your knees into your chest. Inhale as you lean forward into the solid foundation of your arms and engage the interior spaces of your pelvis to lift your body off the floor (see fig. 9.17). Use every muscle you have to do this lift, because each part of the body is responsible for lifting itself. Press strongly into your arms, engage your legs, draw your abdomen farther in, squeeze your rib cage, press into your fingertips, and activate your transverse abdominal muscles. Make your breath long, slow, steady, and deep. Ignore the temptation to quicken or shorten your breath. Stay in this lift for ten breaths or more, even if you have to come down and raise back up again.

If you cannot raise your pelvis off the ground, simply raise your knees into your chest and push your arms into the ground. Even if you feel that nothing is happening, this static strength movement builds the muscle fibers that will one day lift you off the floor. Lean forward into your arms, focus on lifting your pelvis with its own strength, breathe, and have faith. I tried this every day for three months before I could even lift myself an inch off the ground, so keep practicing, and one day your pelvis will come up too. Charging your inner body with energy right before entering final relaxation encourages your entire body to rest completely. Without this powerful charge, some muscles and tissues would not fully release their tension.

After at least ten breaths, jump immediately back into Chaturanga Dandasana rather than coming to rest. Inhale and go into Urdhva Mukha Svanasana; exhale into Adho Mukha Svanasana. Jump forward to standing and chant the closing mantra of Ashtanga Yoga (see Appendix A). Next, inhale and raise your hands as in Surya Namaskara A, exhale and fold forward, inhale and look up, exhale and jump back. Inhale and go into Urdhva Mukha Svanasana, exhale into Adho Mukha Svanasana, and finally jump through to lie down and rest in Sukhasana, or final relaxation (see fig. 9.18).

SUKHASANA

Easy, Comfortable Pose

This pose is often called Savasana in other styles of yoga, but in the Ashtanga Yoga method it is called Sukhasana, or Easy, Comfortable Pose.

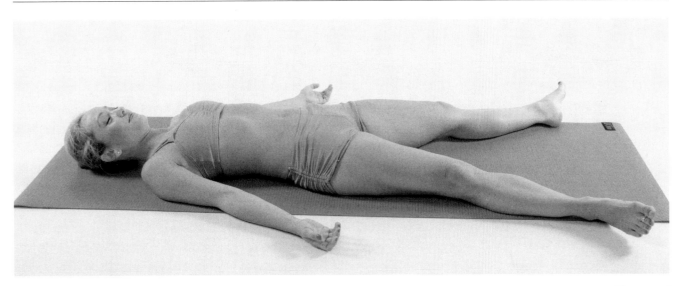

Figure 9.18

In Ashtanga Yoga the posture called Savasana, literally translated as "corpse pose," is a challenging movement in the Fifth Series. Here you should simply lie down and relax.

From Downward-Facing Dog jump through and lie down. Spread your feet wider than hip-width apart and let them externally rotate as much as is natural for you. Relax all the work in your legs. Roll your shoulder blades down your back and spread your arms at approximately the same angle as your legs. Open your shoulders and let the palms turn up. Close your eyes, clear your mind, and stay here for at least five minutes but not longer than twenty minutes. If you have a hard time calming your mind, bring your attention to the breath and the subtle body.

10

Strength: The Yoga of True Power

THE ASHTANGA YOGA METHOD CAN BE THOUGHT OF AS a heroic journey to the center of the soul. Each practitioner faces certain tests and trials along this sacred path. One of the great lessons that each weary traveler of the spiritual path of yoga must learn is the lesson of strength. In Ashtanga Yoga, strength is not measured in mere brute force or physical prowess. Instead, the power and presence demanded by the full yoga practice cultivate a kind of inner fortitude that can only be described as spiritual realization.

Although one of the products of a lifelong commitment to Ashtanga Yoga is a lithe body that is capable of gravity-defying moves, the journey that takes you there is entirely a spiritual one. The process of building the strength and structural support you need to facilitate a healthy range of motion is not an end in itself. Rather, the poses are testing grounds on which you learn liberating life lessons that teach self-esteem, self-confidence, and self-worth. Most people who first attempt to balance on their hands or stand on their head often feel that these poses are impossible for them. When faced with new movements, the mind often rebels and presents a preconceived notion about what the body can and cannot do. Most of these beliefs are deeply entrenched within the individual psyche and are more closely related to emotional boundaries than to any real truth about physical or spiritual potential. On the yoga mat, your deeply held beliefs about yourself become evident, and confronting those beliefs within this safe space can lead to liberation. If you believe yourself to be weak and quit easily, then the challenge of strength will be a good teacher that may take many years to get through to you. If you believe you are naturally strong and will be able to perform the yoga poses easily, strength may teach you humility.

In yoga practice, strength is not just a physical experience, a way to build lean muscle mass. Rather, the strength gained in yoga practice is more about steadying the mind and healing the body. Many people think that yoga is all about flexibility and stretching. While a good portion of it does work on making the body more bendy, the real heart of yoga is a balance between strength and flexibility for the body and mind. Strength in yoga demands a balance between openness and stability. For example, you must have a solid structural foundation in your shoulders so you can bear your body weight while allowing the joints to be free enough for a natural range of motion. Strength in yoga is an integration of the sum of the body, mind, and soul in a way that gives access to something much larger than any individual part.

Once you stand at the bottom of a mountain that feels impossible to climb and then with slow, steady perseverance begin to find the technique, strength, and faith needed to ascend to the peak, you build self-esteem. The challenging arm balance positions in the Ashtanga Yoga method are meant to do just that. The idea in yoga is that there is no one to ultimately rely upon for your success except yourself. When most students attempt the heroic lifts of the Ashtanga Yoga method, they stand at the bottom of their own mountain of impossibility and slowly, steadily begin the humble work of finding their own inner strength. Yoga does not ask you to be strong from the first day. You might not be able to perform various yoga poses on the first try, but if you unroll your mat every day and try for many years, the promise that yoga makes you is that one day you will indeed be strong beyond your wildest dreams. When you see the techniques presented here, you will be challenged and your limits will be tested. This is a good thing! Only if you actually reach your limits will you ever grow spiritually, mentally, or physically.

THE QUIET STRENGTH OF A WOMAN'S BODY

Contemporary dogmas of what is possible for men and women contribute to what yoga practitioners believe is possible for male and female bodies. If you are a woman, you may wonder whether you are the wrong shape, size, weight, or gender to be able to catapult your hips through the air and resign yourself to being just flexible. But this type of thinking undermines a true sense of power for either gender.

In yoga, there is an unfair assumption that all men effortlessly perform gravity-defying lifts and all women snake their way into positions a contortionist would envy. While the mind-set of teachers and students often perpetuates some traditional gender roles, reality tells a different story. There are men who are hypermobile and unable to lift their butts off the ground, and there are women who are stiff as a board but can balance unwaveringly in a handstand. One of yoga's greatest lessons is that there are no universal standards for bodies and that all bodies, genders, races, and ages can benefit from and master this ancient practice.

When you look for evidence that women can be strong in the yoga world, you dig into the very essence of femininity. Sometimes it seems like women who can perform asanas that require great strength are overcompensating, being tough to excel in a male-dominated world. Locking down traits typically associated with femininity, such as softness, openness, sensitivity, and tenderness, means that powerful women are often feared for their harshness.

Trading quintessential female traits to succeed in a man's world devalues women's essence. The complexity of gender is such that there are no easy answers to what constitutes essential male or female traits. My personal journey into yoga led me to ask the difficult question of whether the natural strength in a woman's body is different but not less than a man's. I started out thirteen years ago as the stereotypical, flexible girl with no strength. In awe of the mysterious lift-up, all arm balances, handstands, and vinyasas, I looked critically at the extra cushioning around my bum, small arms, and petite frame and blamed my shape and gender for what I could not do easily. Male teachers in the West meant well and simply let me slide, saying they did not expect women to match men's strength. Movement-based, scientifically backed anatomy books state that women's bodies have a lower center of gravity and therefore work with a different set of rules, casting women as the physically weaker gender. Science, stereotypes, and points of view were creating an artificial limit, so I dug in deeper.

My ninety-three-year-old master Jois once said in a group conference in Mysore, "Yoga is changing. Now some women are very strong. Correct asana performing is possible. Before, not possible. Now possible. All women are doing all asanas correctly." Jois's teacher, Krishnamacharya, was the first Brahmin teacher to allow women into the secret study of the Indian sacred texts and is also quoted as saying that women are the future of yoga. In a world of quickly equalizing power, it is fitting that women's role in yoga also changes and evolves. The basic teaching in yoga is the unification of extremes, and in that light, it is appropriate that both men and women are asked to move toward a balance between strength and flexibility. When I attempted to experience this balance in my own body, I was pushed to the limit of my physical, emotional, and spiritual potential.

BANDHAS

Most people equate physical strength with upper body strength, but Ashtanga Yoga teaches your entire body to be strong from the inside out. Each part is integrated with the larger whole while retaining individual

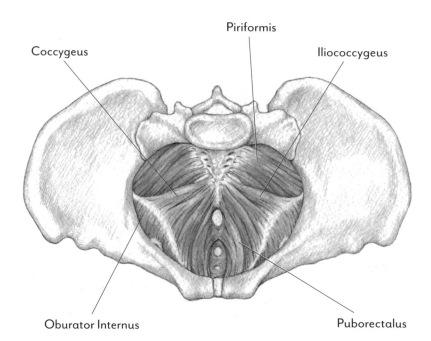

Coccygeus

Piriformis

Iliococcygeus

Oburator Internus

Puborectalus

Figure 10.1

responsibility for lifting, stretching, and strengthening itself. When they try to lift their hips off the ground, many students feel as though their arms are too short, their upper body is too weak, or their bums are too large. The answer to this doubt is the magical mystery of the *bandhas,* which literally means "locks." These mysterious locks are internal and can be cultivated through the careful use of the pelvic muscles. We will discuss the movements that help you feel the bandhas, but remember that these are energetic experiences that are closer to emptiness than to any muscular movement. When you find out just how strong you can be at the center of your body, you will feel light and liberated. The bandhas are invaluable in the sacred effort to bring energy up the spine, along the central column of the body, and through the crown of the head.

Mula Bandha

Root Lock

Sit in a comfortable, cross-legged position on the floor with your spine in a neutral, erect position. Feel both your sit bones and the space between them. Now squeeze your sit bones together without changing the position of your pelvis and without squeezing your gluteal muscles. Next, feel your tailbone and pubic bone. Draw them closer together so that all four points of your pelvis move toward each other. Increase the level of activation so that your sit bones, tailbone, and pubic bone draw in as much as possible. This consciously activates the interior space of your pelvis (see fig. 10.1).

Be careful not to change the position of your pelvis or activate your thighs and gluteal muscles.

Next, contract your anus and squeeze your urethra as though you are stopping yourself from urinating. Add that to the activations you're already doing. Contract your perineum (pelvic floor) by lifting it into your pelvis. If you are a woman, squeeze your cervix and the walls of your vagina; if you are a man, lift your testicles. Connect your anus, urethra, perineum, and genitals in one big contraction. Finally, draw this contraction into your body along your spine and try to move it up and in. Feel the movement into the interior space of the pelvis. Over time you will be able to activate this whole network of movements in one fluid contraction.

Uddiyana Bandha
Upward Flying Lock

Applying what you now know about mula bandha, relax your stomach and let go of any overexertion in your abdominal muscles. Draw your belly, from the navel to the pubic bone, back and into your body as though you are trying to suck in your stomach to fit into a tight pair of jeans. Let this action be released but not soft, more like an elongation than a static contraction. Try thinking about it as a reverse contraction or a sucking in of the abdominal muscles. If the abdominal wall hardens, let go and start again.

Combine the mula bandha action with this reverse contraction, and let all the muscles come together to provide support for your pelvis and lift from within. Breathe into your lungs — into the front, back, and sides of your body — while allowing the energy of the breath to travel up and down your spine. Avoid breathing into your belly; in the challenging movements of Ashtanga Yoga, this can predispose you for injury.

Application

The pelvic floor and the accompanying muscles are like any other part of the body. The more you use them, the stronger they get on a physical and energetic level. You can expect your awareness and control of this area to increase as you practice more. The total contraction in these exercises is intended to help you feel your body. In your yoga practice, you can apply the tools of the bandhas at anywhere from 10 percent to 100 percent of their activation and power. When working on challenging strength poses, you will need every ounce of activation possible. When working on flexibility poses, you will need only a certain percentage of this power to support your spine and pelvis. Activating these muscles is the key to making your pelvis

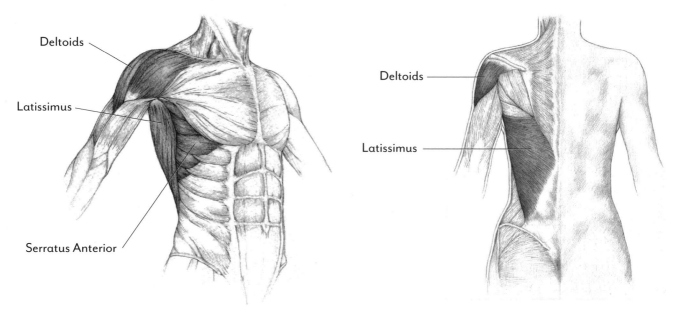

Deltoids

Latissimus

Serratus Anterior

Deltoids

Latissimus

Figure 10.2

Figure 10.3

and hips strong enough to lift themselves from within. Once you literally feel your pelvic floor, you will be able to direct your body through space from the inside out. It is important to be able to connect to the dynamic work of the bandhas in all positions of the spine, through extended, flexed, and neutral poses.

It might be useful to think of mula bandha and uddiyana bandha coming together to create an energetic sensation of emptiness or even brilliant light located at your center of gravity. The spiritual power center inside the pelvis is referred to by some classical Hatha Yoga texts as the Kanda center. All 72,000 nadis are said to originate from this deep place inside the pelvic region. Only by drawing your life energy back to this power center can you actualize the full potential of the Ashtanga Yoga method.

FOUNDATION

The upper body is crucial to the development of strength but works most efficiently when it is integrated into the whole. Rather than thinking about arm strength, it is better to develop a solid structural foundation.

Begin on your hands and knees. Align your shoulders over the palms of your hands and your hips over your knees. Relax your spine. Engage your fingertips, plant your knuckles (but not your fingers or palm), and thrust the heel of your hand into the floor. Allow the "smiles" of your elbows to point approximately forty-five degrees forward and rotate your shoulders down your back to open them. Broaden your collarbones and guide your

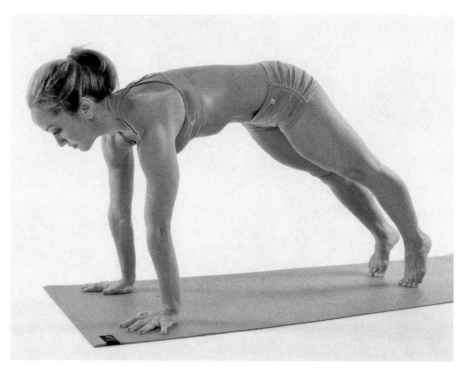

Figure 10.4

shoulder blades down your back and away from each other. Activate your deltoids, latissimus dorsi, and serratus anterior muscles (see figs. 10.2 and 10.3). Lift the center of your sternum to fill out the space between your shoulders. Draw your ribs in, apply mula bandha and uddiyanan bandha, and tuck your tailbone under. Finally, engage your legs and straighten your knees while keeping your chest forward over your hands (see fig. 10.4). This is the foundational position from which all strength-based poses can be performed. If you find it challenging, hold the position for as long as possible once a day and you will grow stronger.

DIRECTION IN STRENGTH

While the external result of strength in yoga means you lift "up" into a headstand, a handstand, or many other arm balances, the truth is that you transfer the weight of your body forward over a solid foundation that integrates your arms with the strength of your torso and the bandhas. When you direct your pelvis over your arms, the magical "up" happens along the way. The great Zen riddle of strength in yoga is that if you think *up,* you will go down, and if you think *forward,* up happens along the way. When working on a headstand, jumping back and through (covered in the next section), Bujapidasana, and other arm balances, find the direction forward with your pelvis over your arms as the foundation to initiate movement.

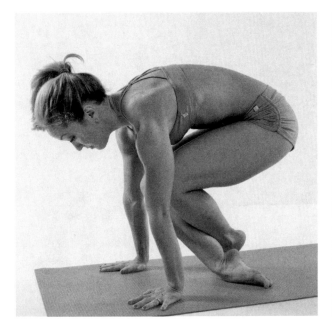

Figure 10.5

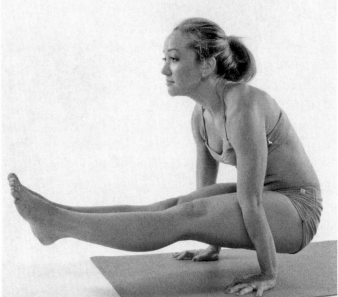

Figure 10.6

HOW TO JUMP THROUGH

When I first tried Ashtanga Yoga, I thought this was one of the most mysterious movements. It looked like magic and seemed impossible. I watched students of all shapes and sizes start in Adho Mukha Svanasana, bend their knees, and float through their arms to come to a sitting position. When I tried it the first time, I nearly hit my arms with my feet and toppled over. But with regular practice, a bit of technique and anatomical knowledge, and the grace of a good teacher, I figured out an easy way to break down this technique so almost anyone can do it.

There are four segments that should ultimately be combined. First, walk or jump your feet forward to a crossed position (see fig. 10.5). Second, guide your feet through your hands by either walking, wiggling, lifting, or sliding them forward while keeping your hands firmly planted on the ground. Third, stretch out your legs so they are extended forward while your hips remain above the ground and your shoulders are strongly engaged (see fig. 10.6). Fourth, complete the movement and lower yourself to a seated position on the ground. Keep your spine in a flexed position throughout the movement.

For the beginner's option, start in Adho Mukha Svanasana and lean your weight forward onto your arms, building a solid foundation in your upper body and strengthening your shoulder girdle. Next, bring your right foot forward so that the top of it rests on the floor behind your hands; point your toes. Keep your pelvis off the ground and your spine flexed.

Bring your left foot forward, point your toes, and cross your left foot behind the right. Your knees should be pointing between your arms. Keep the heels of your hands planted on the ground, your abdomen drawn in, and your pelvic floor engaged. Slowly begin to wiggle your right foot forward a few inches, then repeat the wiggle with the left foot. Keep your hands planted flat on the ground and your hips high. Aim forward with your pelvis and keep your upper body strong. Keep wiggling and inching your way, foot by foot, through your arms until both legs are stretched out in front of you. Lower your hips and pelvis to the floor. Ignore the temptation to rush, lift your hands, or just sit down. Stay strong mentally and physically.

Once this is easy, jump both feet forward and land with your right and left foot crossed behind your hands, knees pointing between your arms, and hips lifted high. Either drag both feet through at the same time, or lift your feet off the ground by leaning farther forward into your arms and drawing your legs into your chest. Finally, stretch your legs all the way out and lower to the ground. Do not lift your hands at any time.

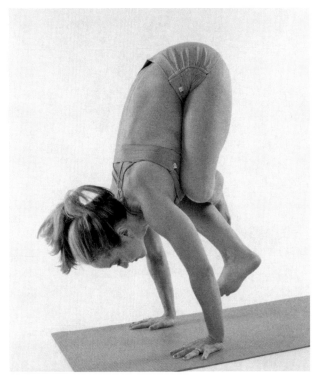

Figure 10.7

The most difficult version of this movement is easy if you have spent enough time performing the beginning versions. Once you are able to walk, drag, or lift your feet through your arms without a problem, you are ready to try for the full jump through. From Adho Mukha Svanasana, bend your knees and look at a spot all the way through your arms. Say to yourself that you will send your hips and pelvis forward over the solid foundation of your arms. Then do it; inhale as you jump forward while pressing firmly into your arms and drawing in your lower belly and rib cage (see fig. 10.7). Keep your legs tucked into your chest and slowly lower them down and through your arms until they are stretched out in front of you. Last, place your hips on the ground. Feel free to combine any version of all these movements as long as you keep breathing throughout your efforts. If you ever feel that your legs can float through your arms without bending, you can jump through with straight legs too.

How to Jump Back

This is one of the most difficult movements in the entire Ashtanga Yoga series. Some students who are able to perform advanced handstands still cannot jump back. The phrase used to describe this movement is a bit misleading, because there is no jump involved. Jumping back is a static lift

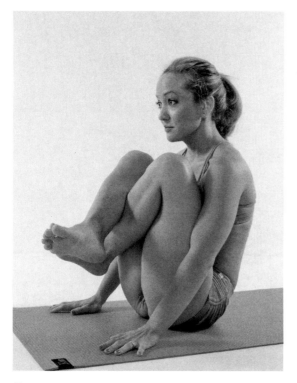

Figure 10.8

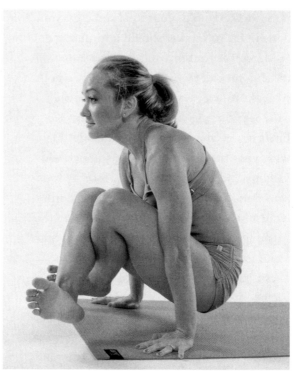

Figure 10.9

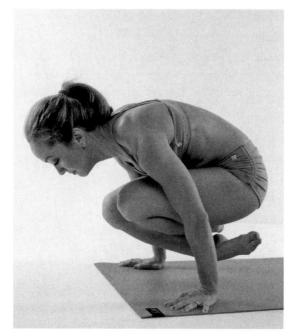

Figure 10.10

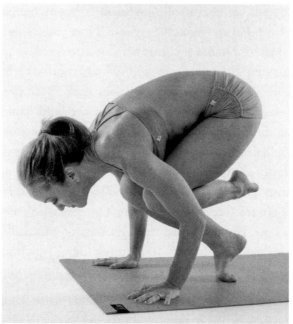

Figure 10.11

with no momentum to help you. Only your strength and understanding of the inner workings of your body will get you through this complex movement.

Starting in any seated pose, begin by crossing your legs into your body as tightly as possible and placing your hands a few inches in front of your hips (see fig. 10.8). This may be challenging, as it involves both a deep external rotation and flexion of the hip joint to get a deep fold and a strong interior space in the pelvis to hold your legs to your chest once they are flexible enough to get there.

Holding your legs against your chest, lean your weight forward onto your hands and allow your pelvis to rise off the ground (see fig. 10.9). Do not worry about up; think about transferring the weight of your body forward onto your arms and hands. Strengthen your shoulder girdle to support this weight, and engage your pelvic floor to lift your hips using their own strength.

If you are a beginner, you will find it impossible to keep your feet off the ground, so slide, wiggle, or walk your feet through your arms as you lean forward, coming into the same position as in the first version (see fig. 10.5). Some rather strong practitioners who are able to lift their feet into this position will get "stuck" halfway back for many years (see fig. 10.10).

Both beginners and advanced students can try the next modification to build strength. With your feet crossed behind your hands, lean forward so that your arms bend and your shoulder girdle strengthens. Then lift one foot off the ground and lean even farther forward, perhaps lowering your head close to the ground as in Chaturanga Dandasana (see fig. 10.11). If you feel your arms shaking and your deltoids and chest muscles burning, be careful not to overdo it, but be aware that this is exactly the strength you need to perform the movement. Finally, allow your legs to either step or float back to Chaturanga Dandasana after you initiate that backward movement by leaning farther forward into your arms.

It took me five years of dedicated practice to learn this movement, and I am still working on improving it. Be patient with yourself and remember to have faith, no matter how hard it seems, that one day you will do it too.

HOW TO JUMP BACK FROM LOTUS POSITION

There are two methods for jumping back from lotus position. The first is to come onto your knees, keeping your legs in lotus (see fig. 10.12). Place your hands in front of your knees, bend your elbows, and push your elbows into your stomach. Lean your weight forward on your hands until

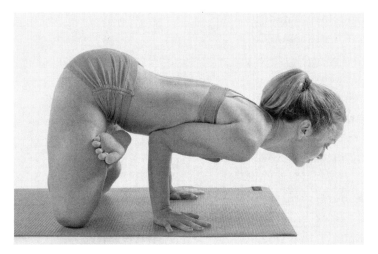

Figure 10.12

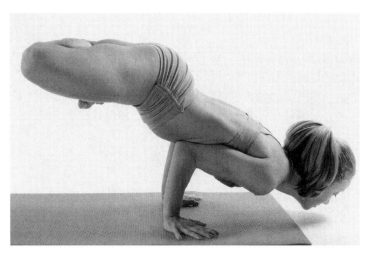

Figure 10.13

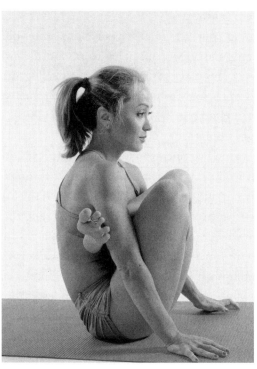

Figure 10.14

your lotus lifts off the ground. When your knees hover in the air, release your lotus, and jump back to Chaturanga Dandasana (see fig. 10.13).

If you are more advanced, lift your lotus position straight off the ground, swing your knees through your arms, and release your lotus to jump back. Hook your feet around your upper arms to get a little extra lift if necessary (see fig. 10.14).

Chakrasana

Wheel Pose

Drishti: Nasagrai (Nose)

Start in a prone position. Place your hands under your shoulders, fingers pointed toward your pelvis. Inhale as you bring your legs over your head.

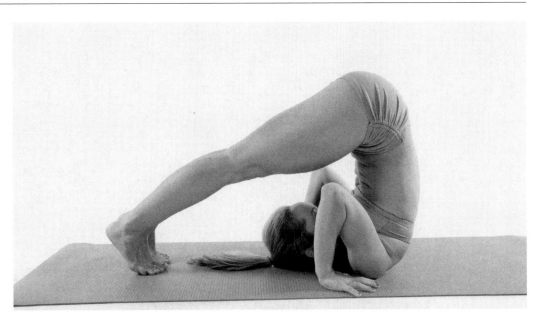

Curl your toes under. Press your hands into the floor as you send your hips over your hands and lift your lower ribs into the core; roll over backward by pressing into your arms (see fig. 10.15). Be sure to inhale as you roll over. Exhale and land in Chaturanga Dandasana.

If you cannot perform the backward roll, try to lift your legs over your head and prepare for the pose. Then rock three times, sending your pelvis over your head while pushing into the floor with your arms and drawing in your abdomen. If you are unsuccessful at this, sit up and jump back normally.

OPENING MANTRA

ॐ

वन्दे गुरूनं चरणारविन्दे सन्दर्शित स्वात्म सुखाव बोधे
निः श्रेयसे जङ्गलिकायमाने संसार हाला हल मोहशांत्यै
आबाहु पुरुषकारं शंखचक्रासि धारिणम्
सहत्र शिरसं शवेतं प्रणमामि पतञ्जलिम

om
vande gurūṇaṁ caraṇāravinde sandarśita svātma sukhāva bodhe |
niḥ śreyase jaṅgalikāyamāne saṁsāra hālā hala mohaśāntyai ||

ābāhu puruṣakāraṁ śaṅkhacakrāsi dhāriṇam |
sahasra śirasaṁ śvetaṁ praṇamāmi patañjalim ||

I bow to the lotus feet of the Gurus
The awakening happiness of one's own Self revealed,
Beyond better, acting like the Jungle physician,
Pacifiying delusion, the poison of Samsara.

Taking the form of a man to the shoulders,
Holding a conch, a discus, and a sword,
One thousand heads white,
To Patanjali, I salute.

CLOSING MANTRA

ॐ

स्वस्तिप्रजाभ्यः परिपालयंतां न्यायेन मार्गेण महीं महीशाः

गोब्राह्मणेभ्यः शुभमस्तु नित्यं लोकाः समस्ताः सुखिनो भवन्तु

ॐ शान्तिः शान्तिः शान्तिः

oṃ
svastiprajābhyaḥ paripālayantāṃ nyāyena mārgeṇa mahiṃ mahiśāḥ |
gobrāhmanebhyaḥ śubhamastu nityaṃ lokāḥ samastāḥ sukhino bhavantu ||
oṃ śāntiḥ śāntiḥ śāntiḥ

May all be well with mankind.
May the leaders of the earth protect in every way by keeping to the right path.

May there be goodness for those who know the earth to be sacred.
May all the worlds be happy.

SŪRYANAMASKĀRAḤ A (9 movements)

EKAM	Inhale, arms up
DVE	Exhale, fold forward
TRĪṆI	Inhale, look up, lengthen
CATVĀRI	Exhale, jump back, Chaturanga
PAÑCA	Inhale, Upward-Facing Dog
ṢAṬ	Exhale, Downward-Facing Dog
SAPTA	Inhale, jump forward, look up, lengthen
AṢṬAU	Exhale, fold forward
NAVA	Inhale, arms up
	Exhale, Samasthiti

SŪRYANAMASKĀRAḤ B (17 movements)

EKAM	Inhale, Utkatasana
DVE	Exhale, fold forward
TRĪṆI	Inhale, look up, lengthen
CATVĀRI	Exhale, jump back, Chaturanga
PAÑCA	Inhale, Upward-Facing Dog
ṢAṬ	Exhale, Downward-Facing Dog
SAPTA	Inhale, right side Virabhadrasana A
AṢṬAU	Exhale, Chaturanga
NAVA	Inhale, Upward-Facing Dog
DAŚA	Exhale, Downward-Facing Dog
EKĀDAŚA	Inhale, left side Virabhadrasana A
DUĀDAŚA	Exhale, Chaturanga
TRAYODAŚA	Inhale, Upward-Facing Dog
CATURDAŚA	Exhale, Downward-Facing Dog
PAÑCADAŚA	Inhale, jump forward, look up, lengthen
ṢOḌAŚA	Exhale, fold forward
SAPTADAŚA	Inhale, Utkatasana
	Exhale, Samasthiti

PĀDĀNGUṢṬHĀSANA (3 movements)
(start with feet apart, hold big toes)

EKAM	Inhale, look up, lengthen
DVE	Exhale, fold forward
TRĪṆI	Inhale, look up, lengthen
	Exhale

PĀDAHASTĀSANA (3 movements)

EKAM	Inhale, hands under feet, look up, lengthen
DVE	Exhale, fold forward
TRĪṆI	Inhale, look up, lengthen
	Exhale, Samasthiti

UTTHITA TRIKOṆĀSANA A (5 movements)

EKAM	Inhale, open to the right, arms out
DVE	Exhale, hold the right big toe
TRĪṆI	Inhale, up
CATVĀRI	Exhale, fold, hold the left big toe
PAÑCA	Inhale, up

UTTHITA TRIKOṆĀSANA B (5 movements)

DVE	Exhale, twist left, hand down
TRĪṆI	Inhale, up
CATVĀRI	Exhale, twist right, hand down
PAÑCA	Inhale, up
	Exhale, Samasthiti

UTTHITA PĀRŚVAKOṆĀSANA A (5 movements)

EKAM	Inhale, open to the right, arms out
DVE	Exhale, right hand down, left arm reaches
TRĪṆI	Inhale, up
CATVĀRI	Exhale, left hand down, right arm reaches
PAÑCA	Inhale, up

UTTHITA PĀRŚVAKOṆĀSANA B (5 movements)

DVE	Exhale, twist left hand down
TRĪṆI	Inhale, up
CATVĀRI	Exhale, twist right hand down
PAÑCA	Inhale, up
	Exhale, Samasthiti

PRASĀRITA PĀDOTTĀNĀSANA A (5 movements)

EKAM	Inhale, open to the right, hands to waist
DVE	Exhale, fold forward, hands on the floor
	Inhale, look up, lengthen
TRĪṆI	Exhale, fold head down
CATVĀRI	Inhale, look up, lengthen
	Exhale
PAÑCA	Inhale, up

PRASĀRITA PĀDOTTĀNĀSANA B (4 movements)

EKAM	Inhale, arms out
DVE	Exhale, hands to waist
	Inhale, look up, lengthen
TRĪṆI	Exhale, fold head down
CATVĀRI	Inhale, up
	Exhale

PRASĀRITA PĀDOTTĀNĀSANA C (4 movements)

EKAM	Inhale, arms out
DVE	Exhale, interlace hands behind back
	Inhale, look up, lengthen
TRĪṆI	Exhale, fold head down
CATVĀRI	Inhale, up
	Exhale

PRASĀRITA PĀDOTTĀNĀSANA D (5 movements)

EKAM	Inhale, hands to waist, look up
DVE	Exhale, fold forward, hold big toes
	Inhale, look up, lengthen
TRĪṆI	Exhale, fold head down
CATVĀRI	Inhale, look up, lengthen
	Exhale
PAÑCA	Inhale, up
	Exhale, Samasthiti

PĀRSVŌTTĀNĀSANA (5 movements)

EKAM	Inhale, open to the right, hands in prayer behind back
DVE	Exhale, fold
TRĪṆI	Inhale, up, turn to the front
CATVĀRI	Exhale, fold
PAÑCA	Inhale, up, open to the side
	Exhale, Samasthiti

UTTHITA HASTA PĀDĀNGUṢṬHĀSANA
(14 movements)

EKAM	Inhale, right leg up, hold toe
DVE	Exhale, fold
TRĪṆI	Inhale, up
CATVĀRI	Exhale, open leg out, look left
PAÑCA	Inhale, leg to the front
ṢAṬ	Exhale, fold
SAPTA	Inhale, up, hands to waist
	Exhale, Samasthiti
AṢṬAU	Inhale, left leg up, hold toe
NAVA	Exhale, fold
DAŚA	Inhale, up
EKĀDAŚA	Exhale, open leg out, look right
DUĀDAŚA	Inhale, leg to the front
TRAYODAŚA	Exhale, fold
CATURDAŚA	Inhale, up, hands to waist
	Exhale, Samasthiti

ARDHA BADDHA PADMOTTĀNĀSANA
(9 movements)

EKAM	Inhale, right foot up, bind
DVE	Exhale, fold
TRĪṆI	Inhale, look up, lengthen
	Exhale
CATVĀRI	Inhale, up
PAÑCA	Exhale, leg down
ṢAṬ	Inhale, left foot up, bind
SAPTA	Exhale, fold
AṢṬAU	Inhale, look up, lengthen
	Exhale
NAVA	Inhale, up
	Exhale, Samasthiti

UTKAṬĀSANA (11 movements)

EKAM	Inhale, arms up
DVE	Exhale, fold forward
TRĪṆI	Inhale, look up, lengthen
CATVĀRI	Exhale, jump back, Chaturanga
PAÑCA	Inhale, Upward-Facing Dog
ṢAṬ	Exhale, Downward-Facing Dog
SAPTA	Inhale, jump forward, Utkatasana
	Exhale, fold forward
AṢṬAU	Inhale, up
NAVA	Exhale, jump back, Chaturanga
DAŚA	Inhale, Upward-Facing Dog
EKĀDAŚA	Exhale, Downward-Facing Dog

VĪRABHADRĀSANA A & B (14 movements)

SAPTA	Inhale, right side Virabhadrasana A
AṢṬAU	Exhale, left side Virabhadrasana A
NAVA	Inhale, right side Virabhadrasana B
DAŚA	Exhale, left side Virabhadrasana B
	Exhale, hands down
EKĀDAŚA	Inhale, up
DUĀDAŚA	Exhale, Chaturanga
TRAYODAŚA	Inhale, Upward-Facing Dog
CATURDAŚA	Exhale, Downward-Facing Dog

PASCHIMATĀNĀSANA A (14 movements)

SAPTA	Inhale, jump through Dandasana (5 breaths)
	Exhale
AṢṬAU	Inhale, hold toes (A), look up
NAVA	Exhale, fold
DAŚA	Inhale, look up, lengthen
	Exhale
AṢṬAU	Inhale, take your wrist (D), look up
NAVA	Exhale, fold
DAŚA	Inhale, look up, lengthen
	Exhale
EKĀDAŚA	Inhale, lift up
DUĀDAŚA	Exhale, jump back, Chaturanga
TRAYODAŚA	Inhale, Upward-Facing Dog
CATURDAŚA	Exhale, Downward-Facing Dog

PŪRVATĀNĀSANA (13 movements)

SAPTA	Inhale, jump through
	Exhale, hands on the floor behinds hips
AṢṬAU	Inhale, up
NAVA	Exhale, down
DAŚA	Inhale, lift up
EKĀDAŚA	Exhale, jump back, Chaturanga
DUĀDAŚA	Inhale, Upward-Facing Dog
TRAYODAŚA	Exhale, Downward-Facing Dog

ARDHA BADDHA PADMA PASCHIMATĀNĀSANA (20 movements)

SAPTA	Inhale, jump through, right foot bind
AṢṬAU	Exhale, fold
NAVA	Inhale, look up
	Exhale
DAŚA	Inhale, lift up
EKĀDAŚA	Exhale, jump back, Chaturanga
DUĀDAŚA	Inhale, Upward-Facing Dog

TRAYODAŚA	Exhale, Downward-Facing Dog
CATURDAŚA	Inhale, jump through, left foot bind
PAÑCADAŚA	Exhale, fold
ṢOḌAŚA	Inhale, look up
	Exhale
SAPTADAŚA	Inhale, lift up
AṢṬAUDAŚA	Exhale, jump back, Chaturanga
EKUNAVIMŚATIḤ	Inhale, Upward-Facing Dog
VIMŚATIḤ	Exhale, Downward-Facing Dog

TIRYANGMUKHAIKAPĀDA PASCHIMATĀNĀSANA (20 movements)

SAPTA	Inhale, jump through, right knee forward
AṢṬAU	Exhale, fold
NAVA	Inhale, look up
	Exhale
DAŚA	Inhale, lift up
EKĀDAŚA	Exhale, jump back, Chaturanga
DUĀDAŚA	Inhale, Upward-Facing Dog
TRAYODAŚA	Exhale, Downward-Facing Dog
CATURDAŚA	Inhale, jump through, left knee forward
PAÑCADAŚA	Exhale, fold
ṢOḌAŚA	Inhale, look up
	Exhale
SAPTADAŚA	Inhale, lift up
AṢṬAUDAŚA	Exhale, jump back, Chaturanga
EKUNAVIMŚATIḤ	Inhale, Upward-Facing Dog
VIMŚATIḤ	Exhale, Downward-Facing Dog

JĀNU ŚĪRṢĀSANA A (20 movements)

SAPTA	Inhale, jump through, right foot in
AṢṬAU	Exhale, fold
NAVA	Inhale, look up
	Exhale
DAŚA	Inhale, lift up
EKĀDAŚA	Exhale, jump back, Chaturanga
DUĀDAŚA	Inhale, Upward-Facing Dog
TRAYODAŚA	Exhale, Downward-Facing Dog
CATURDAŚA	Inhale, jump through, left foot in
PAÑCADAŚA	Exhale, fold
ṢOḌAŚA	Inhale, look up
	Exhale
SAPTADAŚA	Inhale, lift up
AṢṬAUDAŚA	Exhale, jump back, Chaturanga
EKUNAVIMŚATIḤ	Inhale, Upward-Facing Dog
VIMŚATIḤ	Exhale, Downward-Facing Dog

JĀNU ŚĪRṢĀSANA B (20 movements)

SAPTA	Inhale, jump through, right foot in
AṢṬAU	Exhale, fold
NAVA	Inhale, look up
	Exhale
DAŚA	Inhale, lift up
EKĀDAŚA	Exhale, jump back, Chaturanga
DUĀDAŚA	Inhale, Upward-Facing Dog
TRAYODAŚA	Exhale, Downward-Facing Dog
CATURDAŚA	Inhale, jump through, left foot in
PAÑCADAŚA	Exhale, fold
ṢOḌAŚA	Inhale, look up
	Exhale
SAPTADAŚA	Inhale, lift up
AṢṬAUDAŚA	Exhale, jump back, Chaturanga
EKUNAVIMŚATIḤ	Inhale, Upward-Facing Dog
VIMŚATIḤ	Exhale, Downward-Facing Dog

JĀNU ŚĪRṢĀSANA C (20 movements)

SAPTA	Inhale, jump through, right foot in
AṢṬAU	Exhale, fold
NAVA	Inhale, look up
	Exhale
DAŚA	Inhale, lift up
EKĀDAŚA	Exhale, jump back, Chaturanga
DUĀDAŚA	Inhale, Upward-Facing Dog
TRAYODAŚA	Exhale, Downward-Facing Dog
CATURDAŚA	Inhale, jump through, left foot in
PAÑCADAŚA	Exhale, fold
ṢOḌAŚA	Inhale, look up
	Exhale
SAPTADAŚA	Inhale, lift up
AṢṬAUDAŚA	Exhale, jump back, Chaturanga
EKUNAVIMŚATIḤ	Inhale, Upward-Facing Dog
VIMŚATIḤ	Exhale, Downward-Facing Dog

MARĪCHĀSANA A (20 movements)

SAPTA	Inhale, jump through, right knee up
AṢṬAU	Exhale, fold
NAVA	Inhale, look up
	Exhale
DAŚA	Inhale, lift up
EKĀDAŚA	Exhale, jump back, Chaturanga
DUĀDAŚA	Inhale, Upward-Facing Dog
TRAYODAŚA	Exhale, Downward-Facing Dog

CATURDAŚA	Inhale, jump through, left knee up
PAÑCADAŚA	Exhale, fold
ṢOḌAŚA	Inhale, look up
	Exhale
SAPTADAŚA	Inhale, lift up
AṢṬAUDAŚA	Exhale, jump back, Chaturanga
EKUNAVIMŚATIḤ	Inhale, Upward-Facing Dog
VIMŚATIḤ	Exhale, Downward-Facing Dog

MARĪCHĀSANA B (20 movements)

SAPTA	Inhale, jump through, left foot in, right knee up, bind
AṢṬAU	Exhale, fold
NAVA	Inhale, look up
	Exhale
DAŚA	Inhale, lift up
EKĀDAŚA	Exhale, jump back, Chaturanga
DUĀDAŚA	Inhale, Upward-Facing Dog
TRAYODAŚA	Exhale, Downward-Facing Dog
CATURDAŚA	Inhale, jump through, right foot in, left knee up, bind
PAÑCADAŚA	Exhale, fold
ṢOḌAŚA	Inhale, look up
	Exhale
SAPTADAŚA	Inhale, lift up
AṢṬAUDAŚA	Exhale, jump back, Chaturanga
EKUNAVIMŚATIḤ	Inhale, Upward-Facing Dog
VIMŚATIḤ	Exhale, Downward-Facing Dog

MARĪCHĀSANA C (16 movements)

SAPTA	Inhale, jump through
	Exhale, take posture twist to the right
AṢṬAU	Inhale, lift up
NAVA	Exhale, jump back, Chaturanga
DAŚA	Inhale, Upward-Facing Dog
EKĀDAŚA	Exhale, Downward-Facing Dog
DUĀDAŚA	Inhale, jump through
	Exhale, take posture twist to the left
TRAYODAŚA	Inhale, lift up
CATURDAŚA	Exhale, jump back, Chaturanga
PAÑCADAŚA	Inhale, Upward-Facing Dog
ṢOḌAŚA	Exhale, Downward-Facing Dog

MARĪCHĀSANA D (16 movements)

SAPTA	Inhale, jump through
	Exhale, left foot lotus right, knee up, twist right, bind hands
AṢṬAU	Inhale, lift up

NAVA	Exhale, jump back, Chaturanga
DAŚA	Inhale, Upward-Facing Dog
EKĀDAŚA	Exhale, Downward-Facing Dog
DUĀDAŚA	Inhale, jump through
	Exhale, right foot lotus left knee up, twist left, bind hands
TRAYODAŚA	Inhale, lift up
CATURDAŚA	Exhale, jump back, Chaturanga
PAÑCADAŚA	Inhale, Upward-Facing Dog
ṢODAŚA	Exhale, Downward-Facing Dog

NĀVĀSANA (11 movements)

SAPTA	Inhale, jump through, legs up, reach forward
AṢṬAU	Inhale, lift up
	repeat SAPTA ASTAU 5 times
NAVA	Exhale, jump back, Chaturanga
DAŚA	Inhale, Upward-Facing Dog
EKĀDAŚA	Exhale, Downward-Facing Dog

BHUJAPĪḌĀSANA (13 movements)

SAPTA	Inhale, jump around hands, cross feet
AṢṬAU	Exhale, fold chin down
NAVA	Inhale, lift up
	Exhale, Bakasana
DAŚA	Inhale, lift up
EKĀDAŚA	Exhale, jump back, Chaturanga
DUĀDAŚA	Inhale, Upward-Facing Dog
TRAYODAŚA	Exhale, Downward-Facing Dog

SUPTA KŪRMĀSANA (14 movements)

SAPTA	Inhale, jump back, Kurmasana
AṢṬAU	Exhale, take arms back
NAVA	Cross feet
DAŚA	Inhale, lift up with both legs behind the head and look up
	Exhale, Bakasana
EKĀDAŚA	Inhale, lift up
DUĀDAŚA	Exhale, jump back, Chaturanga
TRAYODAŚA	Inhale, Upward-Facing Dog
CATURDAŚA	Exhale, Downward-Facing Dog

GARBHA PIṆḌĀSANA (13 movements)

SAPTA	Inhale, jump through, take Dandasana
AṢṬAU	Exhale, take lotus, arms through, take face
NAVA	Exhale, roll in circles (inhale up, exhale down)

KUKKUṬĀSANA (13 movements)

NAVA	Inhale, lift up, take Kukkuṭāsana
	Exhale, down, release arms
DAŚA	Inhale, lift up
EKĀDAŚA	Exhale, jump back, Chaturanga
DUĀDAŚA	Inhale, Upward-Facing Dog
TRAYODAŚA	Exhale, Downward-Facing Dog

BADDHA KOṆĀSANA (13 movements)

SAPTA	Inhale, jump through, feet together
AṢṬAU	Exhale, fold, chest forward (A)
NAVA	Inhale, up
DAŚA	Exhale, fold, head down (B)
EKĀDAŚA	Inhale, up
	Exhale
DUĀDAŚA	Inhale, lift up
TRAYODAŚA	Exhale, jump back, Chaturanga
CATURDAŚA	Inhale, Upward-Facing Dog
PAÑCADAŚA	Exhale, Downward-Facing Dog

UPAVIṢṬHA KOṆĀSANA (14 movements)

SAPTA	Inhale, jump through, hold feet
AṢṬAU	Exhale, fold
NAVA	Inhale, look up
	Exhale
DAŚA	Inhale, lift up, look up
	Exhale
EKĀDAŚA	Inhale, lift up
DUĀDAŚA	Exhale, jump back, Chaturanga
TRAYODAŚA	Inhale, Upward-Facing Dog
CATURDAŚA	Exhale, Downward-Facing Dog

SUPTA KOṆĀSANA (14 movements)

SAPTA	Inhale, jump through
	Exhale, lie down
AṢṬAU	Inhale, legs up, take toes
NAVA	Inhale, roll up, hold
	Exhale, down
DAŚA	Inhale, look up
	Exhale
EKĀDAŚA	Inhale, lift up
DUĀDAŚA	Exhale, jump back, Chaturanga
TRAYODAŚA	Inhale, Upward-Facing Dog
CATURDAŚA	Exhale, Downward-Facing Dog

SUPTA PĀDĀNGUSṬHĀSANA (26 movements)

SAPTA	Inhale, jump through
	Exhale, lie down
AṢṬAU	Inhale, right leg up, take toe
NAVA	Exhale, fold
DAŚA	Inhale, head down
EKĀDAŚA	Exhale, externally rotate right leg to the side, look left
DUĀDAŚA	Inhale, leg to the front
TRAYODAŚA	Exhale, fold
CATURDAŚA	Inhale, head down only
PAÑCADAŚA	Exhale, leg down
ṢOḌAŚA	Inhale, left leg up, hold toe
SAPTADAŚA	Exhale, fold
AṢṬAUDAŚA	Inhale, head down
EKUNAVIMŚATIḤ	Exhale, externally rotate left leg to the side, look right
VIMŚATIḤ	Inhale, leg to the front
EKĀVIMŚATIḤ	Exhale, fold
DUĀVIMŚATIḤ	Inhale, head down
TRAYOVIMŚATIḤ	Exhale, leg down
CATURVIMŚATIḤ	Inhale, Chakrasana
	Exhale, Chaturanga
PAÑCAVIMŚATIḤ	Inhale, Upward-Facing Dog
ṢAṬVIMŚATIḤ	Exhale, Downward-Facing Dog

UBHAYA PĀDĀNGUSṬHĀSANA (13 movements)

SAPTA	Inhale, jump through
	Exhale, lie down
AṢṬAU	Inhale, legs up
	Exhale, take toes
NAVA	Inhale, roll up, look up
	Exhale, down
DAŚA	Inhale, lift up
EKĀDAŚA	Exhale, jump back, Chaturanga
DUĀDAŚA	Inhale, Upward-Facing Dog
TRAYODAŚA	Exhale, Downward-Facing Dog

ŪRDHVA MUKHA PASCIMATĀNĀSANA (15 movements)

SAPTA	Inhale, jump through
	Exhale, lie down
AṢṬAU	Inhale, legs up
	Exhale, take feet
NAVA	Inhale, roll up, balance with straight arms
DAŚA	Exhale, fold head toward thigh
EKĀDAŚA	Inhale, head up, straight arms
	Exhale, hold the position

DUĀDAŚA	Inhale, lift up
TRAYODAŚA	Exhale, jump back, Chaturanga
CATURDAŚA	Inhale, Upward-Facing Dog
PAÑCADAŚA	Exhale, Downward-Facing Dog

SETU BANDHĀSANA (13 movements)

SAPTA	Inhale, jump through, lie down
AṢṬAU	Exhale, prepare for the pose with feet out, arms crossed
NAVA	Inhale, lift up
DAŚA	Exhale, down
EKĀDAŚA	Inhale, Chakrasana
	Exhale, Chaturanga
DUĀDAŚA	Inhale, Upward-Facing Dog
TRAYODAŚA	Exhale, Downward-Facing Dog

ŪRDHVA DHANURĀSANA (13 movements)

SAPTA	Inhale, jump through, lie down
AṢṬAU	Exhale, prepare
NAVA	Inhale, lift up
DAŚA	Exhale, down
	repeat NAVA DAŚA 3 times
EKĀDAŚA	Inhale, Chakrasana
	Exhale, Chaturanga
DUĀDAŚA	Inhale, Upward-Facing Dog
TRAYODAŚA	Exhale, Downward-Facing Dog

PASCHIMATĀNĀSANA (14 movements)

SAPTA	Inhale, jump through
	Exhale
AṢṬAU	Inhale, hold feet or wrist, look up
NAVA	Exhale, fold
DAŚA	Inhale, look up, lengthen
	Exhale
EKĀDAŚA	Inhale, lift up
DUĀDAŚA	Exhale, jump back, Chaturanga
TRAYODAŚA	Inhale, Upward-Facing Dog
CATURDAŚA	Exhale, Downward-Facing Dog

SARVĀṄGĀSANA (11 movements)

SAPTA	Inhale, jump through
	Exhale, lie down
AṢṬAU	Inhale, lift up

HALĀSANA (11 movements)

AṢṬAU	Exhale, lower feet, bind

KARṆAPĪḌĀSANA (11 movements)

AṢṬAU	Exhale, bend knees, bind

ŪRDHVA PADMĀSANA (12 movements)

NAVA	Inhale, take lotus balance

PIṆḌĀSANA (12 movements)

NAVA	Exhale, fold, bind

MATSYĀSANA (12 movements)

NAVA	Exhale, lift up

UTTĀNA PĀDĀSANA (12 movements)

NAVA	Inhale, take pose
	Exhale, down
DAŚA	Inhale, Chakrasana
	Exhale, Chaturanga
EKĀDAŚA	Inhale, Upward-Facing Dog
DUĀDAŚA	Exhale, Downward-Facing Dog

ŚĪRṢĀSANA (11 movements)

SAPTA	Exhale, prepare
AṢṬAU	Inhale, up
NAVA	Exhale, halfway down
	Inhale, lift up
DAŚA	Exhale, down
	Balasana 5 breaths
EKĀDAŚA	Exhale, jump back, Chaturanga
DUĀDAŚA	Inhale, Upward-Facing Dog
TRAYODAŚA	Exhale, Downward-Facing Dog

BADDHA PADMĀSANA/YOGA MUDRĀ (14 movements)

SAPTA	Inhale, jump through
AṢṬAU	Exhale, take pose
NAVA	Exhale, fold, yoga mudra

PADMĀSANA (14 movements)

DAŚA	Inhale, come up, take pose

UTPLUTIḤ (14 movements)

EKĀDAŚA	Inhale, lift up
DUĀDAŚA	Exhale, jump back, Chaturanga
TRAYODAŚA	Inhale, Upward-Facing Dog
CATURDAŚA	Exhale, Downward-Facing Dog
PAÑCADAŚA	Inhale, jump forward, look up
ṢOḌAŚA	Exhale, fold
	Inhale, Samasthiti
EKAM	Inhale, arms up
DVE	Exhale, fold forward
TRĪṆI	Inhale, look up, lengthen
CATVĀRI	Exhale, jump back, Chaturanga
PAÑCA	Inhale, Upward-Facing Dog
ṢAṬ	Exhale, Downward-Facing Dog
SAPTA	Inhale, jump through, lie down, rest
	Final relaxation

SURYA NAMASKARA A

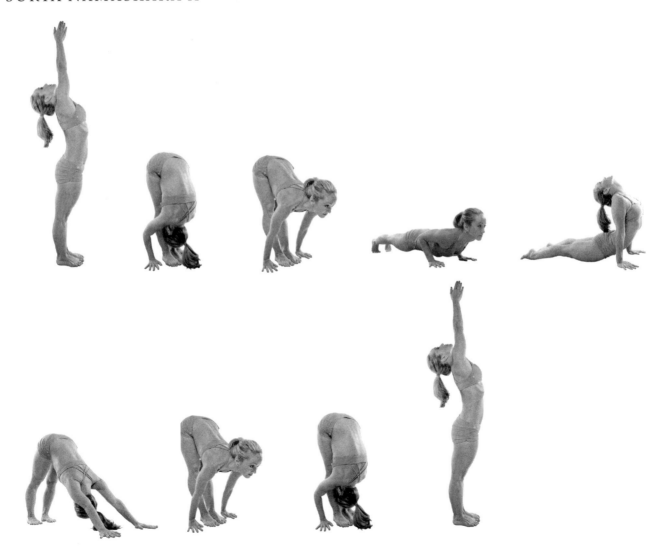

SURYA NAMASKARA B

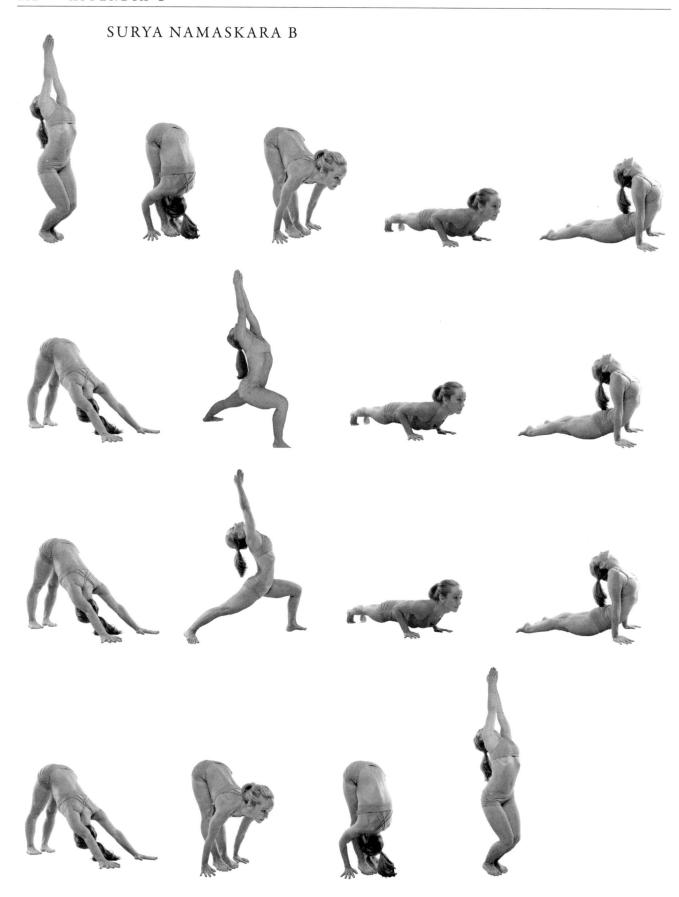

STANDING POSES

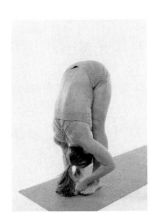

Padangusthasana

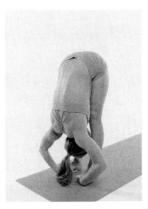

Padahastasana

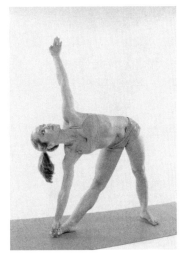

Utthita Trikonasana

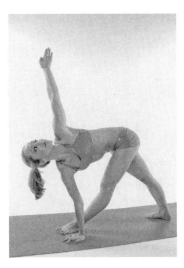

Parivrtta Trikonasana

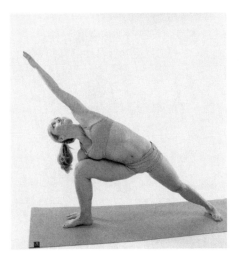

Utthita Parsvakonasana

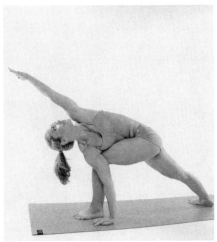

Parivrtta Parsvakonasana

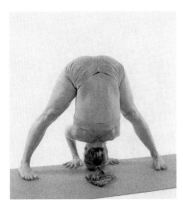

Prasarita Padottanasana A

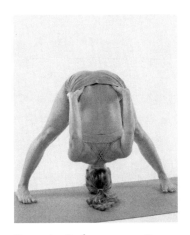

Prasarita Padottanasana B

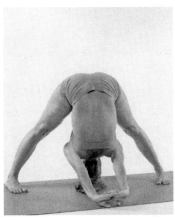

Prasarita Padottanasana C

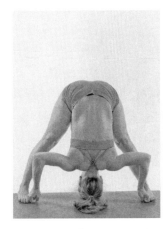

Prasarita Padottanasana D

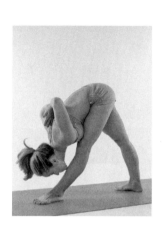

Parsvottanasana

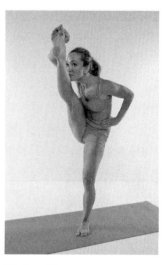

*Utthita Hasta
Padangusthasana A*

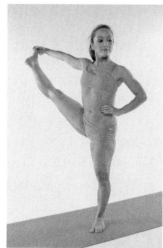

*Utthita Hasta
Padangusthasana B*

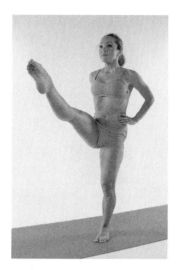

*Utthita Hasta
Padangusthasana C*

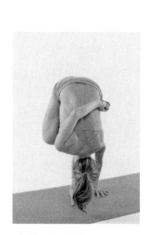

*Ardha Baddha
Padmottanasana*

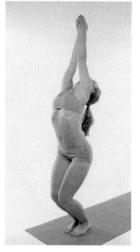

Utkatasana

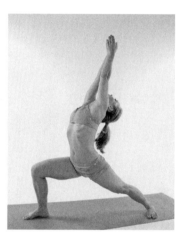

Virabhadrasana A

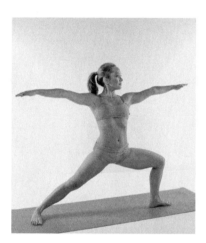

Virabhadrasana B

SEATED POSES

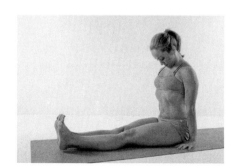

Dandasana

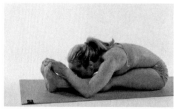

Paschimattanasana A

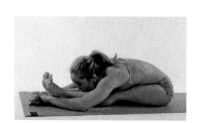

Paschimattanasana D

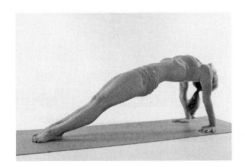

Purvattanasana

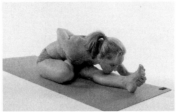

Ardha Baddha Padma Paschimattanasana

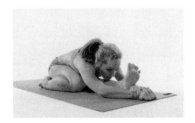

Tiryang Mukha Ekapada Paschimattanasana

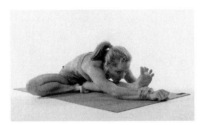

Janu Sirsasana A

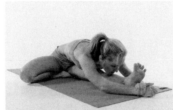

Janu Sirsasana B

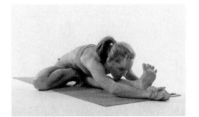

Janu Sirsasana C

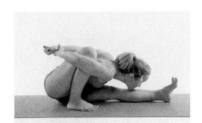

Marichasana A

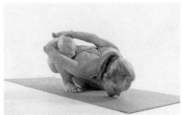

Marichasana B

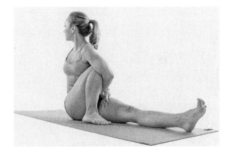

Marichasana C

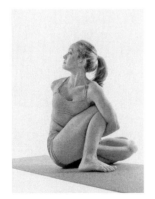

Marichasana D

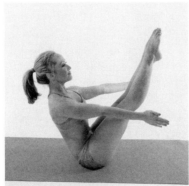

Navasana (five times)

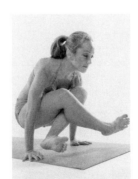

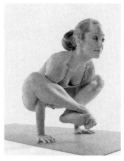 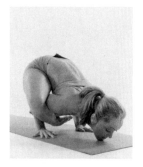 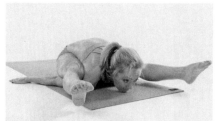 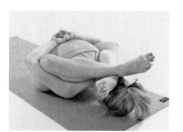

Bhujapidasana   *Kurmasana*   *Supta Kurmasana*

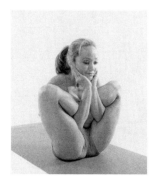 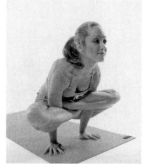 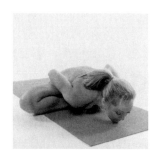 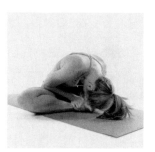

Garbha Pindasana   *Kukkutasana*   *Baddha Konasana A*   *Baddha Konasana B*

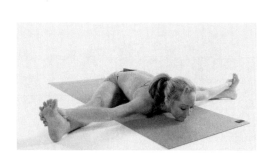 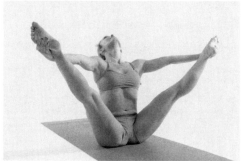

Upavistha Konasana

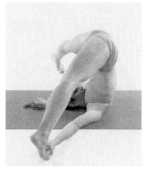 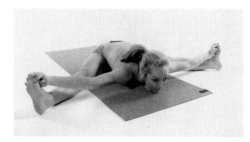

Supta Konasana

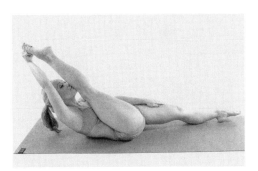

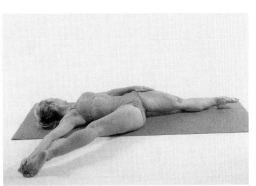

Supta Padangusthasana

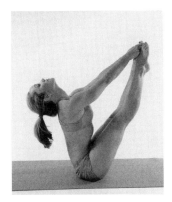

Ubhaya Padangusthasana

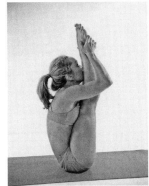

Urdhva Mukha Paschimattanasana

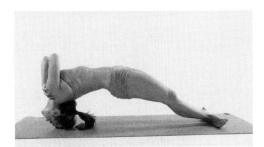

Setu Bandhasana

BACKBENDS

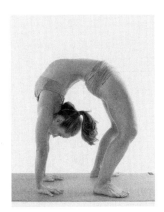

Urdhva Danurasana (three times)

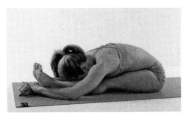

Paschimattanasana

CLOSING POSES

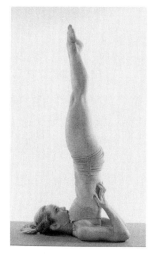

Salamba Sarvangasana

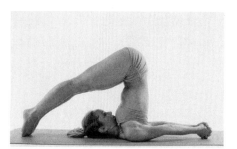

Halasana

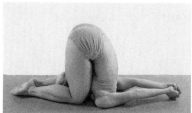

Karnapidasana

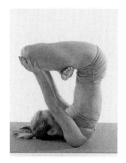

Urdhva Padmasana

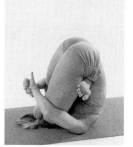

Pindasana

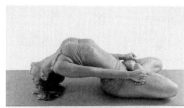

Matsyasana

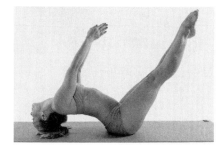

Uttana Padasana

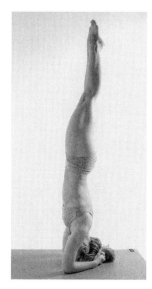

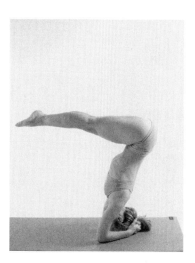

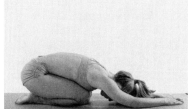

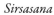

Sirsasana

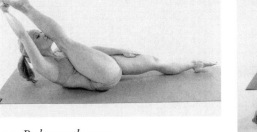

Supta Padangusthasana

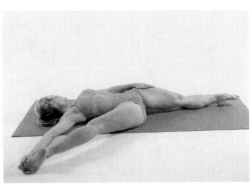

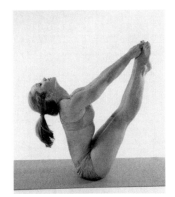

Ubhaya Padangusthasana

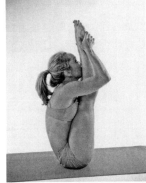

*Urdhva Mukha
Paschimattanasana*

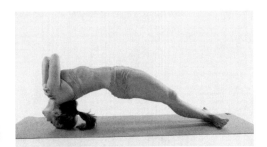

Setu Bandhasana

BACKBENDS

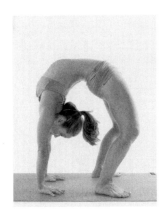

*Urdhva Danurasana
(three times)*

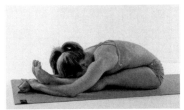

Paschimattanasana

CLOSING POSES

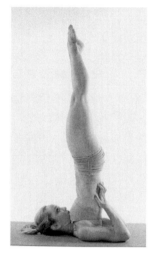

Salamba Sarvangasana

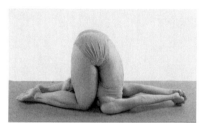

Halasana

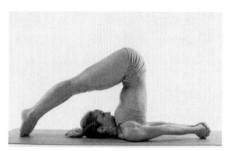

Karnapidasana

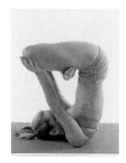

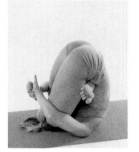

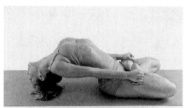

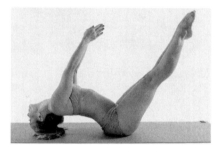

Urdhva Padmasana   *Pindasana*   *Matsyasana*   *Uttana Padasana*

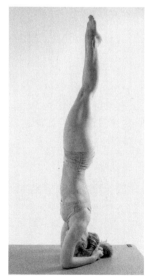

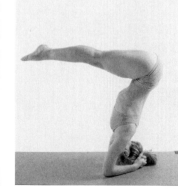

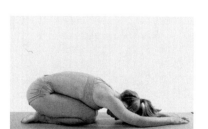

Sirsasana

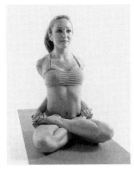
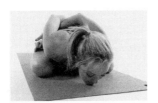
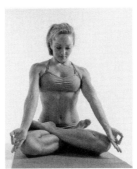
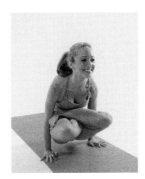

Baddha Padmasana   *Yoga Mudra*   *Padmasana*   *Utplutih*

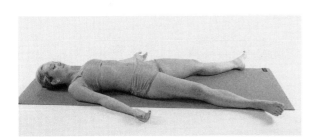

Sukhasana

ADVAITA VEDANTA: The philosophy following the spiritual tradition of the Vedas that believes in the fundamental truth of nonduality, or the ultimate connection between the individual self and the highest, divine Self.

AGNI: Sanskrit for "fire," also represented by the Hindu deity Agni.

AHAMKARA: One of the three components of citta, symbolizing the ego.

AHIMSA: The first of the yamas on the eight-limbed path of Ashtanga Yoga, literally "nonviolence."

ANANDAMAYA KOSHA: The innermost, rarefied of the five koshas, the bliss body, associated with samadhi.

ANNAMAYA KOSHA: The outer layer of the koshas, associated with food, sometimes called the Food Body.

APARIGRAHA: Nonattachment or nonpossessiveness, the fifth of the yamas in Patanjali's Yoga Sutras.

ASHTANGA YOGA (also called Ashtanga Vinyasa Yoga): The eight-limbed path of yoga devised by Patajali; more specifically the system of yoga propagated by the late Sri K. Pattabhi Jois that combines Patanjali's Yoga Sutras, the classical Hatha Yoga poses, and philosophy with the Bhagavad Gita into a total system of spiritual transformation.

ASTEYA: Nonstealing, the third of the yamas in Patanjali's Yoga Sutras.

ATMAN: The true, eternal self that transcends time and space.

AYURVEDA: Indian system of medicine translated as the "science of life"; Sri K. Pattabhi Jois strongly recommended following Ayurvedic principles for yoga practitioners.

BANDHA: Sanskrit for "lock," referring to the three energetic locks in the body — mula bandha, uddiyana bandha, and jalandhara bandha.

BHAGAVAD GITA: Key selection from the Mahabharata epic on the eve of the great battle of Kurukhsetra where Krishna as the avatar of God gives the warrior prince Arjuna the teaching of yoga, sometimes given the status of an Upanishad.

BRAHMA GRANTHI: The karmic knot associated with Brahma that lies at the sacrum along the central energy channel of the body.

BRAHMACHARYA: The restraint of sexual impulses, the fourth of the yamas in Patanjali's Yoga Sutras.

BRAHMAN: The one singular universal divinity, the supreme God.

BUDDHI: One of the three components of citta, signifying the higher intelligence and the source of wisdom and discriminative discernment.

CHAKRAS: Translated as "wheels," energy centers along the subtle body; there are seven main chakras in the human energy system, starting at the base of the spine and ending at the top of the head.

CITTA: Often taken to mean the mind, it is comprised of three components: ahamkara, buddhi, and manas. It includes the subconscious mind and the full flow of consciousness.

DHARANA: Concentration, the sixth limb of the eight-limbed path of Ashtanga Yoga in Patanjali's Yoga Sutras.

DHRIK-STHITI: Stability of vision, being able to control the flow of the energy intake from the sense organs, absolute concentration on a single point of attention.

DHYANA: Meditation, the seventh limb of the eight-limbed path of Ashtanga Yoga in Patanjali's Yoga Sutras.

DIVYA DEHA: The divine body, the goal of all Hatha Yoga practice.

DRISHTI: The gazing point stipulated in each pose utilized in Ashtanga Yoga as taught by Sri K. Pattabhi Jois to train the mind to be singular and strong; one of the components of the Tristana method of Ashtanga Yoga.

EKAGRATA: One-pointedness, the ability to maintain the mind on a single chosen object of attention for a sustained period of time.

GRANTHI: Energetic and karmic knots that lie along the central column of the innermost body, which must be purified and burned through with yogic practice.

GUNA: Sanskrit for "strand" or "chord," referring to the three gunas (sattva, rajas, tamas) in which Prakriti takes manifestation.

Bryant, Edwin. *The Yoga Sutras of Patanjali.* New York: North Point Press, 2009.

Donahaye, Guy, and Eddie Stern. *Guruji: A Portrait of Sri K. Pattabhi Jois through the Eyes of His Students.* New York: North Point Press, 2012.

Feuerstein, Georg. *The Deeper Dimension of Yoga: Theory and Practice.* Boston: Shambhala Publications, 2003.

Frawley, David. *Yoga and Ayurveda: Self-Healing and Self-Realization.* Twin Lakes, Minn.: Lotus Press, 1999.

Freeman, Richard. *The Mirror of Yoga: Awakening the Intelligence of Body and Mind.* Boston: Shambhala Publications, 2012.

Jois, Sri K. Pattabhi. *Yoga Mala: The Original Teachings of Yoga Master Sri K. Pattabhi Jois.* New York: North Point Press, 2010.

Long, Ray. *The Key Muscles of Hatha Yoga: Scientific Keys, Vol. 1.* Baldwinsville, N.Y.: Bandha Yoga Publications, 2005.

Mohan, A. G., and Ganesh Mohan. *Krishnamacharya: His Life and Teachings.* Boston: Shambhala Publications, 2010.

Swami Svatmarama. *Hatha Yoga Pradipika*, 3rd edition. Munger: Bihar School of Yoga, 1998.

Yogananda, Paramahansa. *The Yoga of the Bhagavad Gita.* Los Angeles: Self-Realization Fellowship, 2007.

Videos of the poses in the complete Ashtanga Yoga Primary Series may be found at www.shambhala.com and at the author's Web site www.kinoyoga.com.

UJJAYI PRANAYAMA: The deep breathing practice that forms the basis for the breathing method in the Ashtanga Yoga practice; inhalation and exhalation are vocalized and equal to each other, sometimes reaching up to ten seconds; translated as "the breath of victory."

UPANISHAD: Sacred philosophical texts that form the basis of the orthodox schools of Indian spiritual thought.

VAJRA DEHA: Adamantine body, the body that glows and is strong like a diamond; one of the stated goals of Hatha Yoga practice of asana.

VASANA: An aggregate collection of the individual's samskaras.

VEDAS: Ancient spiritual texts dating to the thirteenth century B.C.E., considered to be divine revelation, consisting of four main works: Rigveda, Yajurveda, Samaveda, and Atharvaveda.

VIJNANAMAYA KOSHA: The second most subtle of the five koshas, symbolizing the body of wisdom, associated with buddhi, close to realization but not the final step.

VINYASA: The coordination of breath with movement that founds the Ashtanga Yoga method; the system of counting each movement in the yoga practice with a Sanskrit number.

VISHNU GRANTHI: One of the three granthis that lie along the sushumna nadi that must be purified through yogic practices; associated with Vishnu and said to be in the heart center.

VIVEKA KHYATIR: Discriminative discernment, one of the stated goals of the eight-limbed path of Ashtanga Yoga in Patanjali's Yoga Sutras; the ability to see and decipher the truth.

VRITTI: Wave or fluctuation appearing on the field of consciousness known as citta; can be both painful and harmless.

YAMA: The first of the eight-limbed path of Ashtanga Yoga in Patanjali's Yoga Sutras comprising moral codes that include ahimsa (nonviolence), satya (truthfulness), asteya (nonstealing), brahmacharya (sexual continence), and aparigraha (nonattachment).

YOGA CHIKITSA: Yoga therapy, also known as the Primary Series of Ashtanga Yoga as taught by Sri K. Pattabhi Jois.

PURUSHA: The eternal, deathless, changeless Self in traditional yoga philosophy, sometimes taken to mean the individual soul or the universal soul.

RAJAS: One of the three gunas, associated with motion, energy, and passion.

RISHI: Seer, usually taken to mean the seer who originally received the Vedas.

RUDRA GRANTHI: One of the three granthis that lie along the sushumna nadi that must be purified through yogic practices; associated with Shiva and said to be in the third eye.

SAMADHI: The last limb of the eight-limbed path of Ashtanga Yoga in Patanjali's Yoga Sutras; the final state of peace.

SAMSKARA: Repetitive behavioral and thought patterns that take root within the citta.

SANTOSHA: Contentment, the second of the niyamas listed in Patanjali's Yoga Sutras.

SATTVA: One of the three gunas, associated with peace, harmony, and balance.

SATYA: Truthfulness, the second of the yamas listed in Patanjali's Yoga Sutras.

SAUCA: Cleanliness, the first of the niyamas listed in Patanjali's Yoga Sutras.

SIX POISONS: Six obstacles that Sri K. Pattabhi Jois said lived around the heart, which must be purified through yogic techniques: anger, desire, greed, sloth, envy, and delusion.

SUBTLE BODY: The body comprised of subtle sensations that are often imperceptible to the untrained mind.

SUSHUMNA NADI: The central nadi running along the central axis of the body, associated with the spinal column; the pathway that the life force (kundalini) must flow up to reach full liberation along the path of yoga.

SVADYAYA: Spiritual self-inquiry, the fourth of the niyamas and the second component of Kriya Yoga in Patanjali's Yoga Sutras; a paradigm of study when reading spiritual texts.

TAMAS: One of the three gunas, associated with ignorance, resistance, and death.

TAPAS: Heat, the third of the niyamas and the first component of Kriya Yoga in Patanjali's Yoga Sutras; associated with the fire of purification cultivated in Ashtanga Yoga.

TRISTANA METHOD: Presented by Sri K. Pattabhi Jois as the foundations of the daily practice in Ashtanga Yoga; comprised of breath (deep breathing with sound based on the ujjayi pranayama), asana (posture), and drishti (gazing point).

MANAS: Sanskrit for "mind," one of the components of citta symbolizing the more mechanical aspects of the mind.

MANOMAYA KOSHA: The third layer of the five koshas, symbolizing the mental body or body of thoughts.

MATSARYA: Sloth, one of the six poisons that Sri K. Pattabhi Jois mentioned live near the heart.

MOHA: Delusion, one of the six poisons that Sri K. Pattabhi Jois mentioned live near the heart.

MULA BANDHA: The root lock, practiced by engaging the pelvic floor, the practice of which awakens kundalini at the base of the spine.

MYSORE STYLE: The style of Ashtanga Yoga practice, named after the city of Mysore in South India where Sri K. Pattabhi Jois lived, in which students memorize the poses and go at their own pace awaiting help from the teacher only when necessary.

NADI: Energy channels running through the subtle body that yoga purifies, 72,000 mentioned in Classical Hatha Yoga texts.

NADI SHODHANA: Nadi or nerve cleansing, both associated with the Intermediate Series of Ashtanga Yoga and alternate nostril breathing exercises.

NAULI KRIYA: An intense purification exercise stipulated in the Hatha Yoga Pradipika that involves sucking in the lower abdomen and churning the stomach from side to side.

NETI KRIYA: Nasal-cleansing technique mentioned in the Hatha Yoga Pradipika that involves the use of water to cleanse the sinus cavity.

NIYAMA: The second of the eight-limbed path of Ashtanga Yoga in Patanjali's Yoga Sutras; it lists five moral observances for how to treat yourself in accordance with yogic principles.

PRAKRITI: Nature, the eternally changeable manifest world of mind and matter, comprised of the three gunas.

PRANA VAYU: The winds of the life force that, through yogic practices such as pranayama, can be manipulated and controlled.

PRANAMAYA KOSHA: The second most gross of the five koshas, symbolizing the body of energy and air.

PRANAYAMA: Breathing exercises that purify the body in classical yogic practice; also the fourth limb of the eight-limbed path of Ashtanga Yoga in Patanjali's Yoga Sutras.

PRATYAHARA: Sense control by withdrawing the focus of the sense on the external world and drawing their awareness into the innermost body; also the fifth limb of the eight-limbed path of Ashtanga Yoga.

HATHA YOGA PRADIPIKA: Classical Hatha Yoga text written approximately five hundred years ago that contains key teachings on asana, pranayama, bandhas, and other yogic practices.

ISHVARA PRANIDHANA: Devotion to God, included as the third aspect of Kriya Yoga and as the fifth niyama in Patanjali's Yoga Sutras.

JALANDHARA BANDHA: The throat lock, where the chin is placed in contact with the sternoclavicular joint.

JANA DIPTIR: Sanskrit for "the lamp of knowledge," referring to the light that dispels the darkness once the inner work of the Ashtanga Yoga method is complete.

KAMA: Desire, one of the six poisons that Sri K. Pattabhi Jois mentioned live near the heart.

KARMA: The cycle of cause and effect, continuing on a large scale over infinite time.

KARMA ASAYA: The sum total of all karmas remaining and accumulated over multiple lifetimes.

KOSHA: Body, referring to the five koshas of layers that comprise a living being.

KRIYA: Yogic purification practice taken to eradicate obstacles on the physical, mental, or emotional level.

KRODHA: Anger, one of the six poisons that Sri K. Pattabhi Jois mentioned live near the heart.

KUNDALINI: The life force that lies dormant, coiled like a snake at the base of the spine, and that yogic practices seek to awaken and draw up along the central axis of the body to the top of the head.

KUNDALINI SHAKTI: The conception of the life force as a female energy that upon rising to the crown of the head unites with the Supreme Being as the aspirant, then achieves full spiritual realization.

LOBHA: Greed, one of the six poisons that Sri K. Pattabhi Jois mentioned live near the heart.

MADA: Envy, one of the six poisons that Sri K. Pattabhi Jois mentioned live near the heart.

MAHABHARATA: The longest Sanskrit epic poem chronicling the battle between the evil Kauravas and the good Pandavas, contains the yogic teaching of the Bhagavad Gita.

MAHAVRTAM: The great vow, referring to the yamas and niyamas in Patanjali's Yoga Sutras from which no one is excused regardless of class, race, gender, or time.